MEDICAL

HOMŒOPATHY

Steve Smith BA (Hons.) LCH MARH FSDSHom

This book is dedicated to Top Wife

. . . still top after all these years

Winter Press
16 Stambourne Way
West Wickham
Kent BR4 9NF

medhom@winterpress.net

Published by Winter Press, 2007
Originally published South Downs Publishing Company, 2005

ISBN(13) 9781874581901

Printed by Biddles

This book is presented as a collection of natural remedies and as an aid in understanding their use. It is intended for use by professional homœopaths and not as a replacement for professional consultation or treatment.

CONTENTS

ACKNOWLEDGMENTS

FOR THIS EDITION

It came as a huge and delightful surprise that the first edition of this book sold like hotcakes and I am immensely grateful to Colin & Susan Winter for taking up the reins and making sure that it was not only republished but considerably improved upon. Doubtless canonisation is just a question of time.

FOR THE BOOK

No one has been more important to the final shape of this book than my magnificent editor, Amanda Saurin. Without her help, advice and support I would have given up long ago and returned to a life of contented idleness. She has been absolutely fantastic – guiding me gently towards a style that is considerably less colloquial than usual. It is her we must thank for the lack of swear words in this book. It is Amanda who has also made sure that this book is on track and that it got printed at all. No thanks can ever convey my gratitude.

I gave early chapters of this book to several people to read and comment on. The advice and constructive criticism proved absolutely invaluable. I therefore owe huge thanks to Karin Mont, Ian Watson, and Martin Miles. Three people who are way too busy to spend time on me, and yet did so with good hearts. Thank you all – I have changed the whole thing round…hope you like it.

FOR INSPIRATION

When I started my homoeopathy training, I was amazed and inspired by some of the best teachers in this (or any other) country. I still read and refer to the notes I made back then (with my quill and parchment) … and I'm still inspired. So thanks to:

Ian Watson	who taught me that homoeopathy can be simple
Barbara Harwood	who brought show-business into homoeopathy
Robert Davidson	who changed my view of the world
Tony Hurley	who showed us how to understand a remedy
Mike Bridger	who showed how to analyse a case
David Mundy	who brought laughter to the party
Martin Miles	who pushes the boundaries still
Robin Murphy	who inspired a whole generation of students
Kate Diamantopoulo	for my nerves of steel
Pema Sanders	who made me take a case properly
Maggie Lee	who helped me to teach

FOR SUPPORT

Naturally I have been a grumpy bear whilst writing this book, so that means that friends and family have suffered along with me (it seems only fair.) A whole host of people have offered support throughout the process, and I am profoundly grateful. Thanks for the interest and advice to Mo (Top Wife), Paul & Gerry, my mum, dad, and sister, Pete Ladd who awarded me an honorary doctorate long before publication, Ken (I finally did it – now you have to buy a copy), Russ, Clive, and Jem for the beer – it really helped…although not with the spelling, and Yvonne and Richard (Yvonne especially for her advice on eyes.) I also owe an enormous debt to generations of students who have sat through my interminable lectures on medical sciences. It's not over yet – I'll be testing you later!

INTRODUCTION

My intention in writing this book is to provide practitioners and students alike with an easy and accessible reference tool. Having taught medical sciences in several Colleges of Homœopathy over the last 10 years, it has become apparent that there is no text that effectively bridges the homœopathic and medical divide – that is the purpose of this book. As you work your way through each chapter, there are a few brief notes on the anatomy and physiology of the system (in the form of a quick recap.) You'll notice that there are no pictures – there are thousands of resources in other places with fabulous 3-D, full colour, even animated pictures, so I recommend you search them out to refer to alongside this text. My aim has been to simplify the typical disease processes that occur within each system.

The advantage of this approach is that the book can be used as an instant reference for students and practitioners of homœopathy. Every chapter clearly places conventional medical terminology, diagnoses, and treatment within a homœopathic context, whilst also collating the very best specific and therapeutic homœopathic remedies within a medical framework. The remedies and adjunctive treatments laid out here are culled from my own clinical experience and that of those of the busiest and most successful practitioners in the homœopathic world.

How this book works

For ease of reference I have divided the human body into systems - Cardiovascular, Musculoskeletal, Nervous System, and so forth. Each of these systems forms the basis of a separate chapter. Each chapter is broken down in the same way, which is discussed further below:

- Recap of anatomy and physiology
- Pathology
- Conventional treatment
- Homœopathic treatment including specifics and therapeutics
- Where necessary, adjunctive treatment

Thus, if a patient comes to see you suffering from conjunctivitis for example, you can immediately turn to the chapter on the visual system, remind yourself of the relevant anatomy and physiology, look at the conventional treatment they are likely to have been offered, and then examine the homœopathic specifics and therapeutics.

OVERVIEWS OF ANATOMY AND PHYSIOLOGY

Most sections begin with a little bit of a 'memory jogger' covering the anatomy and physiology of that system. These are by no means exhaustive, and those with an interest in the detail of the body's function will probably want to delve deeper. I have included several excellent resources in the 'Preparatory Reading' section.

PATHOLOGY

This is where homœopathy meets medical sciences – our patients turn up with a disease, and frequently with a clear diagnosis. This section explains what these diagnoses mean, and sometimes how they are arrived at. Most pathologies will be accompanied by the typical signs and symptoms of the disease.

Diseases are usually discussed in simple, fairly basic terms – I have tried to keep the information straightforward and plain. I have sometimes added in the cause of the disease; in these instances I am referring to the cause as proposed by our colleagues in the conventional medical world, allowing homœopathic philosophy to take a back seat for a while.

CONVENTIONAL TREATMENT

It may seem rather unorthodox to include a section on conventional treatment in a homœopathic book, but I would contend that it is very important – by understanding what a diagnosis means, what the conventional treatment options are and to recognise where a patient is in terms of their conventional treatment, both the homœopath and patient are empowered.

If our patients are using conventional medicine (as is often the case) then homœopathy is not their alternative medicine – it is their complementary. It seems to me that if the patient is not 'operating in isolation' then neither should we.

In this book I have decided to use conventional terms when discussing conventional medicine. This doesn't always sit easily with homœopathic philosophy but in this instance it seems appropriate. So when, in this section, you see the terms diagnosis, prognosis and side effects, it's important to understand that these terms apply to the allopathic approach. It is highly likely that the same disease will have a different prognosis from a homœopathic perspective, but it seems reasonable to inform the reader of each perspective separately.

HOMŒOPATHIC TREATMENT

Many diseases will have a specific list (or table) of remedies that are suitable for that condition. Often I will suggest some ways to help you choose which remedy is the most appropriate. I do not wish to imply that this 'short-cut' homœopathy is the only (or even the best) way to practice. I believe that careful, well-considered constitutional homœopathy is the height of our craft; no other approach has the depth of action or length of impact. Nevertheless the constitutional approach can be slow, and it is notoriously difficult to master. Additionally, some diseases demand a rapid response from homœopathy; if the patient doesn't get results, they abandon the process, and often become a member of the small (but vociferous) group who say, "I tried homœopathy … it didn't work."

There are some homœopaths who are philosophically opposed to using specific or therapeutic remedies, but in my experience – and these are the three key words – I have seen, day after day, week after week, and month after month that giving a remedy suited to the disease (as opposed to one that is suited to 'the whole person') can have a dramatic and rapid effect.

My approach, at least initially, is to concentrate on what the patient has identified as the most important symptoms they want cured. Once they experience success with homœopathy they are more willing to explore other, more subtle aspects of their case. But it often takes a significant improvement in their physical symptoms (their presenting pathology) to give them (and us) the breathing space to work on more subtle matters.

The remedies mentioned in this book fall into several categories – as follows:

SPECIFICS AND THERAPEUTICS

These are remedies that have worked before in similar circumstances, that have been shown by clinical experience to have a rapid effect on a particular pathology. The most famous example in homœopathy is probably *Arnica* for trauma situations. Many of the tables are lists of specifics. These lists have been drawn from the work of respected homœopaths and from my own clinical experience.

Often within the lists or tables I have given clear differentials. These usually comprise quick and simple ways to choose from a list of a few remedies … basic remedy information (specific to the pathology in question) along with remedy keynotes and modalities. Sometimes this is referred to as "Differential homœopathy", or "Therapeutics."

None of the lists are exhaustive – there are rarely more than a dozen remedies, often less. It is typical that every homœopath constructs his or her own lists. This can take years of being in practice – the remedies I'm giving are simply a starting point.

AFFINITIES

As each system is discussed it will become clear that some remedies that are useful within a particular system crop up again and again – these are 'the usual suspects' – remedies whose action is known to have an affinity with a particular part or system of the body. A classic example would be *Rhus tox*, which has an affinity for the musculoskeletal system. It can be priceless in practice to have a 'toolkit' of a dozen or so remedies for each system, it makes the decision process highly efficient, which can be a great benefit to practitioner and patient alike.

ADJUNCTIVE TREATMENT

In a few pathologies or systems I have included a little adjunctive advice, usually in terms of diet and exercise that experience has shown to be helpful. Along with the doubtless benefits that accrue from looking at adjunctive treatment, I sometimes suspect that patients get better in a shorter time if they are participating in the process. Changing aspects of their diet or their exercise routine encourages them to become an active part of the healing process.

ABBREVIATIONS AND CONVENTIONS

There are only a couple of frequently used abbreviations in this book they are:

< which means worse for

> which means better for

SRP which stands for Strange, Rare and Peculiar (in relation to a symptom)

Most of the remedy names however, have been abbreviated … the full botanical or chemical names of the remedies have a resonance and a poetic beauty all their own. In this book I have used the common argot of the homœopath and homœopathic student. As this is a practical reference book it seemed appropriate to use the names we commonly use in practice.

FINALLY

My hope for this book is that it will get dirty, scruffy, written in, and generally dog-eared from overuse. It is intended as a working tool and as a useful, comprehensive reference. My belief is that homœopathy can be a relatively simple craft, and my aspiration is that this book will make it easier still. Now go and heal the sick.

Steve Smith

September 2007

PREPARATORY AND ACCOMPANYING READING

I have deliberately designed this book so that it can be read without any preparatory work. However, as I said in the Introduction, there is a general assumption throughout the book that anatomy and physiology has been studied. Either system by system (as the book is laid out) or in its entirety.

The books I use as an accompaniment to the lectures on which this volume is based are:

Wynn Kapit & Lawrence M Elson **The Anatomy Colouring Book**

Benjamin Cummings Publishing

ISBN 0-8053-5086-1

Wynn Kapit & Lawrence M Elson **The Physiology Colouring Book**

Harper and Row Publishers, New York

ISBN 0-06-043479-1

I think that it is really important to have a good Medical Encyclopaedia or Dictionary. I use these two, but anything of quality will do.

Peter Wingate **The Penguin Medical Encyclopedia**

Penguin Books

ISBN 0-14-051220-9

Elizabeth A Martin (Editor) **Concise Medical Dictionary**

Oxford University Press

ISBN 0-19-281991-7

For those who demand the very best and most thorough medical reference I suggest The Merck Manual, however it is **very** thorough, and most non-medical people will need a dictionary by their side to make it through the text.

Mark H Beers and Robert Berkow (Editors)

The Merck Manual of Diagnosis and Therapy

Merck Research Laboratories *ISBN 0911910-10-7*

Although I will be making reference to conventional medication, its effects and side effects, it is well worth having a dedicated work as well. I use:

John A Henry (Editor) **The New Guide to Medicine and Drugs**

Dorling Kindersley

ISBN 0-7513-0444-1

It is also assumed that the reader will have a working knowledge of how to use a homœopathic repertory and materia medica, my choices are shown below:

Robin Murphy N.D. **Homeopathic Medical Repertory**

Hahnemann Academy of North America

ISBN 0-9635764-0-2

(I use the second edition of this priceless work, and any page references relate to that version specifically.)

Robin Murphy N.D **Lotus Materia Medica**

Lotus Star Academy

ISBN 0-9635764-0-2

NEW MEDIA

There are a wealth of CD-ROMs, and DVD's available that focus on the anatomy and physiology of the human body. Although many of them are designed for children, this doesn't make them any less useful for our purposes – the hip bone is connected to the thigh bone no matter what age you are, and for some people this is the best way to learn. I recommend the following:

The Ultimate Human Body 2.0 CD ROM

Dorling Kindersley

ASIN: B00004UAAP (ASIN Numbers are Amazon Standard Item Numbers)

Essential Anatomy and Physiology CD ROM

Essential Training Solutions

ASIN: B0006MTTJ0

The Human Body DVD

BBC Worldwide

ASIN: B00005JHYO

Of course there are thousands of web sites to choose from, and surfing will produce some crackers along with dozens of dead ends. Here are a few that I have found useful:

www.merck.com

This site has a number of online texts, including the Merck Manual and some really good graphics, videos and texts about the human body. A really good resource.

www.nhsdirect.nhs.uk

Excellent source of information about the disease process as viewed by conventional practitioners.

www.medicalstudent.com

An enormous resource centre that links to free anatomy, physiology, and pathology information.

www.innerbody.com

Subtitled 'Human Anatomy Online' this site does exactly what it says on the tin. Simple but very effective.

CONTENTS

The musculoskeletal system can be a particularly daunting area to study. With the body containing more than 650 individual muscles and over 200 bones there's a lot to remember. In my experience the homœopathic profession is, on the whole, pretty hopeless when it comes to naming muscles, muscle groups, or bone structures. Our colleagues in other disciplines (reflexologists, aromatherpists, and especially the 'hands on' therapies) are much better educated.

It seems that there is, however, a pretty good argument for not even trying to cram in the name and location of every bone and muscle (although this is a laudable aim) as long as you know where to look for the information when you need it. I would recommend a good, up-to-date anatomy and physiology book; something that you can easily reference and whose style suits you. Some of these textbooks can be rather inscrutable for homœopaths, especially if they are targeted at those with a more thorough grounding.

However, it is important to have a clear grasp of the processes of bone formation and to be clear about our definitions of the components of the musculoskeletal system. So I will cover those aspects, naming all the muscles and bones is for other books and other people.

THE SKELETAL SYSTEM

Bone is the exceptionally hard and dense connective tissue that forms the skeleton of the body. It's composed of a matrix of fibres (collagen fibres) that are impregnated with bone salts. The salts are of importance to us as homœopaths as they correspond to the remedies *Calcarea carbonica* and *Calcarea phosphorica*, remedies which are of great importance in skeletal disorders. Bones also contain small traces of fluoride and magnesium.

The skeleton begins to form in the womb and is initially constructed of only cartilage. By month six mineralisation starts and calcium is taken from the mother's blood, and if necessary from her bones too. As children grow the bones elongate; the growth point being just below the end of the bone (the epiphysis). It is at the epiphysis that large quantities of osteoblasts are engaged in producing new bone, which is later hardened by ossification with the deposit of minerals. It isn't uncommon to hear of a 'slipped epiphysis'; this is when a child has fractured the epiphysis and it has not been correctly realigned, thus causing crooked growth. It should be remembered that bone is a living tissue and consequently in a constant state of flux. Its constituents are constantly being deposited and removed.

Three types of cells perform the regulation of the living bone; Osteoblasts, Osteocytes and Osteoclasts. These cells create, preserve and destroy the bone respectively.

- Osteoblasts are continually building up new bone (and are therefore at their most active in childhood).
- Osteocytes are the cells which are 'left behind' to act as caretakers for the bone. They are capable of detecting stress or fracture and can summon the Osteoblasts back again to undertake any necessary repair.
- Osteoclasts are responsible for removing any unwanted bone.

Obviously these three have to work in some harmony and if there are disturbances to their functioning, then diseases of bone can occur.

Despite common belief to the contrary, bone is an active tissue, which is forming and remodelling constantly in response to the physical stresses and structural demands placed upon the body. At sites of continued excess pressure or traction the bone will form overgrowth, thus creating bone spurs or osteophytes. With chronic joint inflammation or hormonal/mineral imbalance bone will lose substance and increase in brittleness – causing osteoporosis.

CURVATURE OF THE SPINE

Curvatures of the spine mainly occur in one of two ways. The normal curvature of the spine (from the 'front' of the body to the 'rear' – technically anterior to posterior) can be exaggerated; this is called a Kyphosis. Perhaps the most familiar condition associated with this type of spinal curvature is hunchback. This is a humped condition of the dorsal spine resulting from an extreme curvature of the spine.

As a result of the spinal deformity in hunchback, the ribs become contorted, compressing or displacing the lungs and other structures within the chest cavity and thrusting the collarbone and shoulder blades into distorted positions. Deformities take place in the hips and other parts of the body in its effort to maintain balance. So one can see a systemic pathology, which is traceable to a particular problem.

The spine can also deform laterally (side to side) causing a curvature known as Scoliosis. Sometimes the spine deforms twice forming an 'S' shape; this is known as a double scoliosis. Scoliosis is sometimes addressed surgically by insertion of a metal rod along the spine. In some cases the spine twists in both the lateral and posterior planes; perhaps inevitably this is called Kyphoscoliosis.

SPINAL COLLAPSE

Collapse may occur in elderly people, particularly women, whose bones can become soft and brittle, causing a dorsal kyphosis. When curvature results from collapsed vertebrae, the person loses height along with developing the curvature.

CONVENTIONAL TREATMENT FOR CURVATURE OF THE SPINE

Treatment for a hunchback condition is varied. A mild kyphosis can often be corrected with plaster casts and braces if diagnosed before the skeletal frame has completed its growth. It is said that congenital deformities cannot be cured; only a certain amount of the deformity can be minimised by surgery and local manipulation. Hunchback caused by spinal disease is also only slightly amenable to surgery and local treatment. Traction, pads, and plaster-jacket supports are commonly used in manipulative treatments. Conventional medicine asserts that there is no cure for many spinal conditions, and certainly it may be difficult to change such deep pathology. However, there are a number of things that can be done to improve the situation. As usual exercise and homœopathy often combine well to help, and physical complementary therapies are often wonderfully effective; chiropractic manipulation, osteopathy, reflexology and good massage can be life-changing.

EXERCISE

Use it or lose it. Gentle exercise should be beneficial, possibly the best option being Tai Chi. This slow, controlled form of the martial arts is intended to release blocked energy in the body and may indeed help increase flexibility. It also enables people in pain and discomfort to do something with minimal discomfort.

HOMŒOPATHIC TREATMENT

As usual there can be no substitute for a well-indicated constitutional remedy, and if the curvature is congenital, then you need to look carefully at the miasmatic background. However these are the specific remedies worth considering… if in doubt check Murphy's Repertory; Diseases, Spinal curvature, (p.439). [SRP, below = Strange, Rare and Peculiar]

Remedy	Comments
Asafoetida	Syphilitic, extremely sensitive. SRP > cold wet weather.
Calc fluor	< rest, change of weather. > heat and warmth.
Calc phos	Soreness of back as if broken, stiff, cold and numb.
Hecla lava	Tumours, caries of bone, enlarged glands.
Merc corrosivus	< evenings, night, acids. > while at rest.
Phos ac	< exertion, being talked to. > warmth. Scraping pains.

PAGET'S DISEASE

This is a disorder of the normal balance between creation and destruction of bone. In Paget's Disease it is the osteoblasts that are in error in that they are creating more bone than is actually needed and also creating it in an irregular fashion. For the forgetful, osteoblasts are the cells that are responsible for bone formation; osteoclasts are those that remove unwanted bone; and osteocytes are the "caretaker" cells which detect fractures or stress and summon back the osteoblasts (which usually disappear after childhood). This extra creation of cells means that large cavities are produced. These cavities can be filled with vascular fibrous tissue (and consequently with blood). The effort required to circulate the increased volume of blood may lead to heart failure.

SIGNS AND SYMPTOMS

Early symptoms of Paget's disease include bone pain, joint pain (especially in the back, hips and knees), and headache. Physical signs include enlargement and bowing of the thighs (femurs) and lower legs (tibias), and enlargement of the skull in the area of the forehead.

As the disease progresses, other signs and symptoms often appear. These may include further bowing of the affected limbs, a waddling manner of walking, muscle and sensory disturbances, and hearing loss. Congestive heart failure (high-output) may occur. Tumours of the bone (osteogenic sarcoma) are also a rare complication. Most cases of Paget's disease however, are without symptoms and are mild. These may be identified through x-rays of the pelvis. When symptoms occur, they are often vague and hard to distinguish from those of many other bone diseases such as lumbar spine diseases or osteoarthritis.

Diagnosis is confirmed through blood tests – so you need to encourage your patient to get them if you are not sure. X-rays showing characteristic lesions on the back of the head (occiput) and thigh bones (femur) are also important diagnostic findings.

CAUSES

The exact cause of Paget's Disease is not known. Recent scientific research suggests that Paget's disease may be caused by a slow virus. This type of condition involves a virus that may stay dormant in the body for many years, and then reactivate later in life causing disease symptoms. More research is needed to determine whether genetic and/or slow virus factors are involved in the cause of this disorder. It is considered possible by conventional medics that Paget's Disease may have a genetic factor; of course, as homœopaths we feel that all patients have 'genetic factors', consequently this angle should be noted when treating Paget's Disease.

HOMŒOPATHIC TREATMENT

One specific remedy for the condition (under Osteo Deformans in Clarke's Clinical Repertory) is *Hecla lava.* This is a fascinating small remedy and can be studied in Clarke's Dictionary of Materia Medica; Clarke says that one of his acquaintances, when travelling in Iceland, noticed that the sheep in the vicinity of Hecla had immense exostoses (benign cartilaginous outgrowth from a bone) on the jaws.

Clinical experience has shown the power of *Hecla lava* to arrest many forms of bone disease, including osteosarcoma, tubercular bone disease and syphilitic osteitis (inflammation of the bone) and exostoses. Other remedies that may help are *Silica* and *Calc phos*.

RICKETS

These are two names for the same disease; one term (Rickets) refers to the childhood manifestation and the other (Osteomalacia) to the adult manifestation.

Rickets is a nutritional disorder whose manifestation is one of skeletal deformity. It is caused by a decreased mineral concentration in bones and cartilage due to low levels of calcium and phosphorus in the blood. This deficiency is itself traceable to a lack of vitamin D. Vitamin D is essential for the maintenance of normal calcium and phosphorus levels.

The best sources of vitamin D are herring, mackerel, salmon, cheese, and eggs (herring has 10 times more vitamin D than cheese). Vitamin D is leached from the system by lack of sunlight and fried foods.

The type of skeletal deformities depends largely on the child's age when the vitamin D deficiency occurs. A child who has not yet learned to walk develops vertebral curvatures – a walking child develops leg curvatures.

OSTEOMALACIA

This is the adult form of the disease – it obviously doesn't affect growth so much as the mineralisation process. The bones become demineralised. This can be caused by chronic renal failure resulting in loss of calcium from the body or from adult coeliac disease, which prevents calcium from being absorbed.

The disease may well manifest as aching on moving the muscles (as calcium is used in muscle contraction) and spasm in the muscles. A calcium-heavy diet may not prove adequate for the body if it is not being absorbed. One possible solution would be to try prescribing Dolomite, a mineral supplement, which is a mixture of calcium and magnesium (and it is the latter which is often needed for absorption of calcium). Food that is rich in vitamin D is a good plan; as is plenty of sunshine, which is the easiest source.

HOMŒOPATHIC TREATMENT

The table below shows the top five remedies for Osteomalacia; the pattern, which you should be able to spot, is that the most obvious remedies are often a good first choice.

Calcarea carbonica
Silica
Mercury
Calcarea phosphorica
Phosphorus

Any of these remedies may be helpful; either as a constitutional prescription or as a tissue salt to support deeper prescribing. As usual a careful study of the case and knowledge of the remedies should help in the selection process.

PAIN

Pain, understandably, will feature large in practice. Most of our patients will complain of pain of some sort, and in the musculoskeletal system the majority of pathology will have some accompanying pain.

One of the hardest questions for our patients to answer is "What does the pain feel like?" Quite rightly, they often say, "…well it just hurts". But our Materia Medicas and Repertories are highly descriptive of types of pain and how they apply to certain remedies. So it can be worth trying to help the patient to describe the type of pain they are experiencing. It will often be priceless to find out the type of pain our patients are experiencing, so we must train ourselves to have some understanding of the vocabulary of pain. A careful reading of one's repertory, particularly the relevant chapter (for example the chapter on Joints in Murphy's Repertory) can be illuminating.

THE MUSCLES

The human body contains more than 650 individual muscles anchored to the skeleton, which provide pulling power so that you can move around. These muscles constitute about 40% of your total body weight.

Muscles act as pulleys on the levers of bone. Often they function in complementary pairs. Muscles can be strained or pulled – with the typical soreness and ache. When 'irritated' muscles go into spasm. Muscle inflammation can be localised or diffused and muscles can weaken or atrophy – particularly with arthritic joints.

The muscle's points of attachment to bones or other muscles are designated as 'origin' or 'insertion'. The point of origin is the point of attachment to the bone to which the muscle is anchored. The point of insertion is the point of attachment to the bone the muscle moves.

MUSCULAR DYSTROPHY

This is a crippling disease characterised by gradual wasting of skeletal muscle. The clinical course is progressive, with increased weakness and diminution in muscle mass and function until the patient is confined to a wheelchair, remissions do not occur.

CONVENTIONAL TREATMENT

Muscular dystrophy has its origin in a genetic mutation, but the biochemical steps by which this genetic defect manifests itself in the degenerative process in the muscle are not known. Because specific treatment is not available, general measures, including physical and occupational therapy, are used. Genetic tests for mutations in the different genes causing muscular dystrophy provide rapid and accurate diagnosis for patients. In the case of the X-linked Duchenne and Becker muscular dystrophies, these tests allow detection of female carriers of the disorders.

HOMŒOPATHIC TREATMENT

As ever, careful constitutional remedies are probably your best bet – along with (probably) several miasmatic remedies; otherwise look at those in the following table. For good leads in Murphy's Repertory look up Colliquative wasting of body (397) and Muscular Dystrophy (1450).

Remedy	Comments
Antimonium tart	Drowsiness, debility and sweat. < damp, cold > sitting erect.
China	Debility, limb pains. < touch, < after eating, > bent double.
Eupionum	Intense sweat from least exertion. Cramps in calves.
Jaborandi	Profuse salivation, severe sleepiness, excessive sweating.

WHIPLASH

This is one of commonest spinal complaints, a 'motor vehicle based injury' where the head rapidly accelerates and then decelerates, usually due to the sudden arrival of another car in the back seats. The sudden movement of the head primarily affects the neck; the patient suffers from stiffness, pain, headache and any number of concomitants.

CONVENTIONAL TREATMENT

Conventionally clinicians look to support the neck; the focus of the trauma. Often a surgical collar will be used usually allied to some physiotherapy. Medication is also used – most frequently analgesics and muscle relaxants.

HOMŒOPATHIC TREATMENT

Homœopathy can often be seen as a viable complement to conventional treatment. The effects of whiplash can be long lasting, debilitating and difficult to eradicate conventionally. As a consequence of this (and of the alarmingly frequent tendency of cars to biff into each other) we see this complaint quite often in clinic. To find the most pertinent remedies look in Murphy's Repertory in the Neck chapter, (Injuries, whiplash). He places eight remedies in that rubric, here's a quick look at the top four:

HYPERICUM

This remedy is particularly well indicated because it shares the sharp, shooting pains typical of whiplash. It's a good remedy for conditions where the muscles go into spasm (as can happen in whiplash) and also for 'pinched nerves', which can be the underlying pathology in some of these cases.

Patients who need this remedy find their condition to be very painful, and the affected area is very sensitive. They may also experience numbness and tingling – in the case of whiplash this could extend to the fingers and thumbs. So one of the differential indicators for *Hypericum* would be an 'extension' of the syndrome – even if it were just from the neck to the shoulder.

BRYONIA

This is a frequently well-indicated remedy – it is a remedy that has an affinity for the joints (and incidentally for the neck), and in whiplash they are liable to have a 'frozen' neck. These are the people who have to turn their whole body in order to speak to you if you are to one side. They can't just turn their head – their shoulders have to move as well. This remedy is noted for its dryness and this is found in conditions pertaining to the neck as well. The patient may complain of dryness of the neck or, more often, of a 'crunching or grinding' sound when they move their neck. *Bryonia* typically is worse for motion or activity and better for pressure. You will tend to see them applying 'oppositional pressure' where they put the flat of their hand at the point of most pain and 'push against it'. This seems to help a little.

CAUSTICUM

One of the main features of *Causticum* is that they suffer from 'contraction of the muscles'. In the case of whiplash or other neck injury this is likely to be the muscles of one side of the neck, which temporarily contract, giving the patient a distinctive look – with their head leaning off to one side. They also suffer from raw and burning sensations in the muscles and hate to sit in draughts.

RHUS TOX

This is an inevitable choice in any number of musculoskeletal complaints and should be a particularly well-known remedy for first aid treatment. The usual indicators for this remedy here would be great stiffness of the neck and amelioration from heat. Worth thinking of as an excellent remedy for almost any distortion of the spine

FIBROMYALGIA – FMS

First described in 1843 as a type of rheumatism, 'fibrositis' has only recently been recognised as a systemic disorder (like rheumatism itself) with far-reaching effects. It is estimated that 5% of people suffer from fibromyalgia, but the actual figures may well be higher as diagnosis is difficult. There are no specific laboratory tests for fibromyalgia and the symptoms are diverse and vague. People suffering from this may have been on a long and frustrating search for answers and relief. Indeed there will be a preponderance of such people visiting you in practice, because they'll have "tried everything else… might as well try homœopathy". One of the reasons for including fibromyalgia in these pages is because you are likely to be treating this disorder. The medical profession has not been backward in creating synonyms for fibromyalgia; there are a few of them in the table below.

Synonyms for Fibromyalgia
Fibromyositis. Fibrositis
Muscular Rheumatism
Musculoskeletal Pain Syndrome
Nonarticular Rheumatism
Periarticular Fibrositis
Rheumatoid Myositis
Tension Myalgia.

SIGNS AND SYMPTOMS OF FIBROMYALGIA

Patients with fibromyalgia may have a gradual or sudden onset of symptoms. The major symptom of this disorder is muscular pain. Areas that are frequently affected may include muscles in the back of the neck and shoulders, in the low back, the sides of the breastbone, and the bony points of the elbows, hips and knees. In addition, an examining physician will find small specific areas called tender points, which are painful when pressure is applied. Other symptoms found in most patients with Fibromyalgia are: muscle spasms, fatigue, muscle stiffness and non-restorative (unrefreshing) sleep.

Some patients with fibromyalgia may have chest pain, painful periods, difficulty concentrating, headaches, painful and/or frequent urination, diarrhoea, constipation, numbness, dryness in the eyes and mouth, dizziness, swelling of a tendon (tendonitis), swelling of the connective tissue structure surrounding a joint (bursitis), depression and/or anxiety.

The usual suspects for Fibromyalgia remedies are:

Remedy	Comments	Modalities
Cimicifuga	Spasm of large muscles. Twitching and jerking. Sore and bruised all over. Heavy and stiff.	< cold, menses, motion touch. > warmth, pressure
Phytolacca	Inflammation of muscles, fascia, tendons. Sore throats. Shifting changeable pains. Restless, weak, sore all over. Exhausted	< motion, damp, cold, night. > warmth, dryness, rest.
Rhus tox	Connective tissue inflammation. Tearing, drawing, burning. Restless, painful and stiff.	< first motion, rest, cold, damp. > continued motion, warmth, rubbing.
Gelsemium	Heavy, dull, lethargic, aching, numb. Heavy limbs, tired, weak. Loss of muscular power.	< damp, cold, warm wet weather. > urination.
Bryonia	Hardness of painful muscle groups. Headache, fever, heat, swelling. Stitching pain, irritable, thirsty.	< least motion of any part, touch. > rest, lying down, pressure.
Kalmia	Rapidly shifting location. Shooting neuralgic pains. Inflammation.	< motion, touch, cold, left side. > warmth and rest.
Causticum	Chronic inflammation with contraction. Stiffness. Tearing, drawing pains.	< motion, cold clear weather. > warmth, warm bed.

Other muscle disorders that you are likely to encounter commonly include the following:

CRAMP

Cramp occurs where muscles protest over having insufficient blood supply or overuse. *Magnesium phos* and *Colocynth* are good remedies to think of, but there are many that will do just as well.

SPRAIN

This is where the ligament is left stretched and swollen. Treating sprains is more common in some practices than others, often the 'common' first aid remedies (such as *Arnica, Rhus tox, Ruta,* and *Bryonia*) are effective. If in doubt look first at the more obvious remedies.

RSI

Repetitive Strain Injury is increasingly common, now that so many people spend a large part of their working day hunkered down over a keyboard. You won't find the condition in Murphy's Repertory specifically, but if you ignore the 'label' it should be easy to treat… if in doubt, for immediate effect try *Arnica* (it's a trauma injury that's why) and *Rhus Tox* (again the obvious remedies).

PARALYSIS

Which, to be honest, may be a nerve disorder rather than a muscle disorder (e.g. MS). Again there are a cluster of remedies that crop up in this sort of condition, namely *Conium, Causticum, Gelsemium, Phosphorus* and so forth. In cases of paralysis you need to be sure of the pathology and of the aetiology (as the latter may point you to a suitable remedy).

TREATMENT FOR GENERAL MUSCLE DISORDERS

- Exercise: Is absolutely crucial, patients will often benefit from a tailor-made programme created by an expert in the field. "Use it or lose it" is as true of muscle as it is of bone.
- Diet: Plenty of protein – try nuts, pulses, whole grains, seeds (sunflower, pumpkin, etc.), sprouted seeds, fish, fowl, meat and of course, dairy produce.
- Vitamins: Vitamin E, 400 to 1000 International Units daily may be helpful.

HOMŒOPATHIC TREATMENT

Most commonly you will have to deal with acute trauma to the muscles – sprains, strains, overuse, injury and so on. The presenting complaint will be pain or "an ache" in the muscles. It may not be possible for us as homœopaths to distinguish between a muscle strain and a trauma to the tendon. In practise, because the tendon is much less vascular it will take longer to heal… not much help until afterwards, or if your patient already has a diagnosis.

Don't forget that the body will heal itself if given sufficient rest, and that the reverse is also true. Overexertion will often bring the trauma galloping back. Many of your greatest successes will be in treating acute trauma. This is because a) it is easy and b) because people will remember how you made the pain go away. And this is a very powerful memory.

Here are a few remedies that might help in trauma:

Remedy	Comments
Arnica	The number one trauma remedy. Try this first in many instances and train your patients to take it prophylacticly. Bruised sore feeling (all over) <rest lying down >motion.
Rhus tox	<rest, beginning to move >continued motion. Number one strains remedy – stiffness or soreness from overlifting etc. <on grasping.
Ruta	Mechanical injuries of bone and periosteum. Dislocations, lameness after sprains. Parts lain on are painful. Strain of eye muscles.
Causticum	Paralytic conditions of single parts. Rawness and soreness. Feeling of tension and shortening of muscles. Restlessness at night, chilliness >damp, wet weather.
Lactis acidum	Rheumatic pains in joints, esp. knees. Trembling of body while walking. Limbs feel cold.

So far we've looked at a couple of specific conditions and remedies that might be appropriate to treat them. Commonly though patients come with a problem that is 'area specific', but with no particular diagnosis or medical 'label'. For instance someone will say, "Well I just have problems with my ankles" or some such.

So it's worth looking at one area of the muscular system in an area-specific way and offer some remedy possibilities too. Inevitably this approach does not allow us to focus on the muscles at the *expense* of the skeleton or vice-versa. Naturally enough we frequently have to look at the problem as a systemic one, which is what happens in practice. But it can be useful to have in mind some remedies whose affinities are for a definite part of the body.

This small diversion looks at the shoulder, its structure, a typical pathology, some remedies and the body 'language' associated with that area. It isn't difficult to apply these specific examinations to any part of the system, especially with the aid of a good anatomy book, a standard medical text, a good repertory, and a fair measure of common sense. If this sort of approach appeals to you, and you'd rather not do the work yourself I would heartily recommend Asa Hershoff's fabulous book *'Homeopathy for musculoskeletal healing'*, which is published by North Atlantic Books. For now though, let's just take a look at the shoulder joint.

THE SHOULDER

The shoulder forms a so-called 'shallow' joint; this is because it is only held to the body by ligaments and the tendons of the 'rotator cuff' group of muscles. As a consequence the shoulder sacrifices stability for flexibility. (In this it is the exact opposite of the hip, which sacrifices flexibility for stability.)

This sacrifice allows us to move our hands and arms freely for carrying, moving heavy objects or pushing, pulling, and manipulating objects. Sadly though the shoulder is the most easily dislocated joint. It's easily sprained either as an acute response to an easily recognisable task (e.g. "Everything was fine until I spent the weekend painting my bedroom") or the shoulder can be strained because of long-term excess… at the end of a busy football season for example.

FROZEN SHOULDER

Because they are almost constantly in use, the ligaments and capsule of the shoulder can be torn and weakened over time. Inflammation of the joint occurs at the same time as inflammation of the bursa and tendon, creating a persistent problem. Chronic inflammation can cause calcium deposits and adhesions in the shoulder, leading to scar tissue that prevents mobility of the shoulder joint. This is also known as Rotator Cuff Syndrome because it is an inflammation of the Rotator Cuff.

It is a painful disorder and is < movement in any direction. It is worth considering a few remedies that may help because those that help this condition may also be beneficial in other joint disorders. The following remedies, consequently, are worthy of consideration:

RHUS TOXICODENDRON

This is one of the great remedies for the musculo-skeletal system (you'll recall that it's one of the remedies that will often help in arthritis). There can be aetiology of overexertion, following which the shoulder stiffens up causes a limit to the normal range of motion (which is a simple definition of frozen shoulder). The condition is generally > heat – look for patients who are using a hot water bottle. They are usually > stretching exercise too; 'mild' frozen shoulder. In 'bad' frozen shoulder, the patient cannot move the shoulder at all – it's locked. This is a useful remedy for body-builders, athletes and so on.

RUTA GRAVEOLENS

As we've seen with spinal injury this is a remedy for dislocation and stiffening. The shoulder feels weak and lame… and lying on it hurts.

SANGUINARIA

With this remedy there is a tendency for the right shoulder to be affected. The patient complains of a deep burning in the shoulder and neck. There is stiffness and a tender sore spot in the shoulder. There will be pain on movement. This is a good remedy for headache and neck complaints with a concomitant of shoulder pain.

FERRUM METALLICUM

To differentiate from *Sanguinaria* (with one question) this tends to be a left-sided remedy. The patient suffers from stiffness, aching, burning, and a general weakness. We can often see blushing and flushing, even at the site of the problem.

THIOSINAMINUM

This is another remedy that can help after overuse of the shoulder. Helpful for carpenters, builders, mechanics and so on. *Thiosinaminum* can break down adhesions and scar tissue. The muscle may have torn and developed scar tissue which limits the movement, and is aggravated when the shoulder is used. It seems to work well when given low and long to remove scar tissue.

BRYONIA ALBA

One of the outstanding characteristics of this remedy it that parts feel dry, so the shoulder feels as if there isn't enough synovial fluid (also seen in knee pathology). Every motion gives stabbing, sticking pain.

BODY LANGUAGE

It can be helpful to see a physical problem in its wider context. Nothing operates in isolation in the body and there is a case to be made for physical problems reflecting a deeper emotional state. This connection can be particularly helpful in homœopathy where we are often looking for a way to treat the whole person.

I wouldn't advocate the pursuit of connections at the expense of doing the simple thing (which often proves to be the most effective), but I would suggest that an understanding of what physical manifestations may represent can sometimes be a bonus in searching for the right remedy. In the case of the shoulder here are some thoughts:

- Shoulders droop with failure
- Shoulders can puff up with pride and accomplishment
- People say that they have a weight on their shoulders
- Broad shoulders express strength and power
- When we give up, or don't know what to do, we shrug our shoulders

CONVENTIONAL TREATMENT

There are two types of drugs commonly used for muscle problems – muscle relaxants, and analgesics. The latter is covered in other parts of this book (because they cover a multitude of sins). For now let's have a look at the muscles relaxants:-

MUSCLE RELAXANTS

These are used to treat the muscle spasm that can come about with an injury – or even for no apparent reason. Spasms are the involuntary, painful contractions of a muscle or a group of muscles that can cause an arm or leg to stiffen, or make it nearly impossible to straighten your back. Muscle spasms can also be brought about by osteo-arthritis – the pain in the affected area triggering abnormal tension in a nearby muscle. Muscle relaxants are also used to treat spasticity, seen in some neurological disorders, MS, and cerebral palsy. If the spasm is a result of direct injury it may well be treated with a non-steroidal anti-inflammatory drug (NSAID) or analgesic, but if the spasm is severe then muscle relaxants are commonly used. One of the reasons for this kind of treatment is that it will often allow physiotherapy to commence at a stage when it would otherwise not be possible. In some instances the relaxant Botulinum toxin will be used to relax muscle spasm in otherwise inaccessible areas such as those around the eye or in the neck.

HOW DO THEY WORK?

Muscle relaxant drugs work in one of three ways:-

- The centrally acting drugs damp down the passage of the nerve signals from the brain and the spinal column, which cause the muscles to contract, thus reducing excessive stimulation of the muscles.
- Drugs such as Dantrolene reduce the sensitivity of the muscles to nerve impulses.
- When injected locally, Botulinum toxin prevents transmission of impulses between muscles and nerves.

Sadly most centrally acting drugs can have a general as well as a specific affect. Therefore they can have a depressive effect on nervous activity. This produces drowsiness, particularly at the beginning of treatment. Too high an initial dose can cause weakness in the muscles.

RISKS AND SPECIAL PRECAUTIONS

The main long-term risk with muscle relaxants is that the body becomes dependant upon them; consequently if the drugs are withdrawn suddenly the stiffness may be worse than before. So you need to be aware of this if you advise your patients to stop taking them! In rare cases drugs like Dantrolene can cause liver damage. Anyone taking this drug should have his or her blood tested regularly to assess liver function. Unless used with great caution Botulinum toxin can paralyse unaffected muscles and might interfere with such functions as speech and swallowing which can be a bit of an inconvenience.

QUICK CASE NOTES – MUSCLE SPASM

A male patient presented on the phone with severe muscle spasm. The spasm was so bad that it literally brought him to his knees. This was very painful, and somewhat embarrassing.

Remedies prescribed were Arnica 200 hourly and Mag phos tissue salt five times per day. The patient was advised to give the treatment twenty-four hours and, if not better, to see his GP.

After twenty-four hours the problem had not improved significantly and the patient was prescribed Ibuprofen and Diazepam by his GP. He sensibly went to see an ostoeopath and was told, to his amazement, that he had dislocated three ribs and was lucky to be moving at all.

Three sessions with the ostoeopath and continued Arnica stopped the spasms. The lesson here is that homœopathy will not always work (at least not unaided). Don't forget to suggest other therapies – even conventional ones if necessary!

THE JOINTS

Although bones and muscles are obviously the two major components of the musculoskeletal system, there are a number of minor divisions, and we should be sure, before moving on, of our definitions.

JOINTS

Joints are the points at which two or more bones are connected; there are a number of different types of joints.

Synarthroses are rigid, immovable joints, such as the connections between the bones of the skull. These immovable joints are held together by actual intergrowth of bone or by strong fibrous cartilage.

Symphyses are slightly movable joints, such as the junction of the bones making up the front of the pelvis. Slightly movable joints are held together by elastic cartilage.

Diarthroses are movable joints, such as the meeting of the bones of the limbs with those of the trunk. Typical movable joints consist of an external layer of fibrous cartilage giving rise to strong ligaments that support the separate bones.

The bones of movable joints are covered with smooth cartilage and are lubricated by a thick fluid, called synovial fluid, produced between the bones in membranous sacs, known as bursae.

The human body has several types of movable joints. Ball-and-socket joints, which allow free movement in all directions, are found in the hip and shoulder. Hinge joints, allowing movement in one plane only, are found in the elbows, knees, and fingers. Pivot joints, permitting rotation only, are found between the first two vertebrae; the head rotates from side to side on a joint of this type called the axis. Gliding joints, in which the surfaces of the bones move a short distance over each other, are found between the various bones of the wrist and ankle.

LIGAMENTS

Ligaments hold joints together and help to guide their movement, (and therefore *limit* the range of movement). Ligaments provide stability and strength. When at rest our joints 'hang by their ligaments' in order that little or no muscle tension is needed. Ligaments get stiff and contracted with under use or joint disease and are a common site of adhesions. (Adhesion has 2 meanings – 1) refers to the **symptom** where two normally separate surfaces are joined and 2) refers to the **name** given to the fibrous connective tissue itself.)

TENDONS

Muscles taper down to fibrous bands called tendons that attach to bones. Tendons and their linings are most noticeable, as is any part of the body, when they become inflamed (as in tendonitis or tenosynovitis). They can also be affected by chronic injury as in chronic shoulder problems. Tendons, at worst, can rupture – and this requires plastic surgery.

CARTILAGE

Articular cartilage is the lining at the end of the bones. It is smooth and glass-like (well, ideally), so it allows a smooth, low-friction joint surface. Because of poor blood supply, injury to the cartilage heals slowly and poorly. Also the surface of the cartilage can become pitted, cracked and brittle – arthritic change. Some cartilage is spongy and elastic and forms a flexible joint – as in the cartilage discs that join vertebrae. The difficulty with this sort of system is that the discs of cartilage are subject to wear and tear, thinning, bulging and fragmentation.

BURSAE

Bursae, as discussed, are fluid filled sacs around the joints, which act as cushions or lubricating pads and (in theory) allow a smooth gliding surface between tendons and bones. In the case of injury the bursae can become inflamed – leading to bursitis, which is a common painful condition of movable joints.

ARTHRITIS

Arthritis is an inflammation of a joint. Over 100 different diseases can produce arthritis. In its most common and troubling forms, arthritis may occur in one or more joints of the body and is usually a long-term condition that may progressively disable and handicap.

Conventional medicine cannot offer any cure but the disease can be controlled. Pain-relieving and anti-inflammatory drugs are used, as well as programs of exercise, rest, heat, and devices to maintain joint motion and function. Aspirin is still one of the drugs most widely used in treating the disease. Severe cases may be treated with gold compounds or the drugs hydroxychloroquine or penicillamine. Using conventional drugs can markedly reduce disability in advanced cases, and surgery is often effective in correcting deformities.

OSTEOARTHRITIS

This is the process referred to when there is a wearing away of the (often) load-bearing cartilage. As the cartilage is worn away the bone cells beneath try to compensate by proliferating and mineralising the bone. This however cracks and synovial fluid squeezes into the cracks. These are known as Geodes and they further weaken the bone. Where the bone is not being worn away irregular swellings called osteophytes 'grow' – these are seen most clearly as Heberden's Nodes. The main symptom of osteoarthritis is pain, which is < cold & damp. The defining difference between osteoarthritis and rheumatoid arthritis is that osteoarthritis is not better for gentle movement.

It is the most common form of arthritis, affecting an estimated 10% – 15% of the population, especially women; it is a usually mild, sometimes painful disease occurring primarily with advancing age, when degenerative changes alter the structure of the joints. Symptoms may be relieved and the condition controlled with drugs, exercises, and other measures, sometimes including orthopaedic surgery. Homœopathy however can have a significant effect in providing effective treatment of osteoarthritis.

RHEUMATOID ARTHRITIS

Rheumatism gets its name from the word rheuma meaning "a flow of morbid humours". It is not uncommon for the beginning of rheumatism to express itself throughout the whole body in the form of flu-like symptoms and aches and pains. The disease can affect any connective tissue and consequently can appear in the joints, vessels, skin, lungs, eyes and lymphoid tissue.

It is by far the most serious, painful, and potentially crippling form of arthritis; it is chronic, is characterised by flare-ups and remissions, and affects mostly women, but can even attack children. Rheumatoid arthritis attacks the joints primarily but may affect supporting connective tissues throughout the body, causing fever, weakness, fatigue, and deformity. The cause is not known, but a hereditary predisposition and an environmental agent, such as a virus are suspected.

There are a number of theories about the origin of RA but it is possible that it is an autoimmune response whereby the body is attacking its own antibodies. The probability is that whatever the cause, it will spread, causing the synovial membranes to thicken and secrete fluid into the joint. This then swells up and becomes tender and stiff.

Later the synovium proliferates and thickens (as opposed to osteoarthritis wherein it slowly vanishes)... to produce a pannus (cloak). If it is not mobilised there is a risk that the joint will be permanently immovable, thus movement is essential but with the development of the pannus, movement becomes reduced and painful – a 'Catch 22' for the patient.

The disease routinely spreads through the body (polyarthritis) although the hands are often the main target. Apart from the hands, the feet are often affected (resulting in a feeling of walking on pebbles) and the knees can suffer from muscle wastage and possibly a cyst (Baker's Cyst), which can then erupt through the back of the knee.

> Of interest to the homœopath is the rubric
> 'Sensation as if little stones were under the heel when treading on it'
> *Aurum, Bromium, Cann-I, Hepar sulph, Lyc, Rhus tox.*
> From the excellent book "Sensations as if -" By Herbert A Roberts MD.

Many other bodily systems can be involved apart from the joints; most frequently there may be subcutaneous nodules that can be seen on the bones of the knees, elbows and shoulders. There may also be anaemia that arises because the marrow is inhibited from taking up iron. Lymph nodes may be enlarged (especially in children) and there can be a drying up of secretions from the salivary and tear glands – Sjogren's Syndrome – that leads to difficulty swallowing and sore inflamed eyes. In some men with RA there is involvement of the pleura, which leads to breathlessness, whilst women are more likely to suffer carpal tunnel syndrome.

CONVENTIONAL TREATMENT – DRUGS

There are three rules which we should adhere to when dealing with patients on drugs:

- NEVER change your patient's medication without reference to their GP.
- Know your subject – get an up-to-date drug reference book (and a BNF or Mimms).
- Use low potencies, frequently and the remedy will work 'through' the drugs.

Many, if not most, patients who come to see you who have a history of joint disorders/arthritis will also have a history of prescribed and non-prescribed medication. You need to have at least some idea of what is likely to be given; its effects and its side effects. So here goes – following the 'three steps to heaven' approach often adopted by conventional practitioners.

STEP ONE – NON-STEROIDAL ANTI-INFLAMMATORY DRUGS

Known commonly as NSAIDs, these drugs are used to relieve pain, stiffness and inflammation. They are widely prescribed for rheumatoid arthritis, osteoarthritis and other rheumatic conditions. They do not (and are not intended to) alter the course of the disease but they reduce inflammation and thence pain and swelling. Consequently they may often be the first line of defence from a conventional point of view, and then added to later on.

In the main NSAIDs are said to be free from serious side effects. However, nausea, indigestion and altered bowel action are relatively common. Aspirin has a higher potential to irritate the stomach than most of the other NSAIDs although occasionally NSAIDs can cause bleeding in the stomach or duodenum. Patients with peptic ulcers should therefore avoid them. NSAIDs are not usually recommended during pregnancy or during breast-feeding. They can also impair blood clotting.

STEP TWO – ANTI-RHEUMATIC DRUGS

Anti-rheumatic (including systemic corticosteroids) drugs are used to relieve the symptoms of pain and stiffness, maintain mobility and prevent deformity. These are drugs that modify, halt or at least slow the underlying disease process. Corticosteroids are often used in this way because they suppress the immune system (and rheumatism is thought to be an auto-immune disease, therefore…). However the suppression of the immune system for a prolonged period of time brings its own problems, such as an inability to deal adequately with otherwise relatively minor illnesses. Also used is Chloroquine, originally used in the treatment of malaria, this drug has the side effect of causing eye damage. Some patients may receive gold-based drugs, which may be given for years. Side effects here include rashes, digestive disturbances, kidney damage and suppressed blood cell production.

STEP THREE – LOCALLY ACTING CORTICOSTEROIDS

Corticosteroids are given by injection for joint disorders when only one or two joints are involved. There are two stated reasons to account for their effectiveness:-

- They block the production of prostaglandins – chemicals responsible for triggering inflammation and pain.
- They depress the accumulation and activity of the white blood cells (that cause inflammation).

Injection obviously concentrates the corticosteroids at the site of the problem. Possible side effects can include indigestion, weight gain, acne, fluid retention, muscle weakness and mood changes. And if that's not enough you can't drink alcohol with them.

HOMŒOPATHIC TREATMENT

Arthritis will be a common complaint in practice and reputations can be made or lost on dealing with the common complaints. If you help a patient's arthritis (or even reduce their pain and stiffness) word about you will spread.

In acute cases you can hope to reduce inflammation, swelling and the pain. With luck you'll spare fragile tissue, nerves and blood vessels from further damage.

In more chronic cases the well-chosen homœopathic remedy can halt the progression of the disease. Deep acting constitutional treatment is capable of altering existing pathology, returning elasticity, flexibility and function to contracted tissue. As ever, constitutional treatment will improve overall immune responses and metabolic health, as well as taking into consideration the mental/emotional condition of the patient.

What follows is a table of some of my favoured remedies for arthritis. Because this is such a common complaint, there are, inevitably, many remedies to choose from so be aware that the remedy your patient needs might not be in this list. In the end you'll have to (as usual) treat each case on its peculiarities.

Remedy	Signs & Symptoms	Modalities
Aconite	Good first remedy. Sudden onset. Shooting tearing pains. Inflammation of the joints. Fever	< Motion, touch, night >Open air, rest
Bryonia	Absolutely hates movement – wants to be perfectly still. Joints red and shiny. Hot & swollen and puffy	<< Motion, touch >Localised heat, firm pressure
Ledum	Ascending arthritis, especially helpful if the small joints are affected, but also knees and ankles. Stiff, swollen and bruised	< Pressure, motion, heat of bed > Cold applications
Rhus tox	Everybody's first aid remedy for arthritis. Stiff, weak, and restless.	< First motion > Continued motion > Heat
Kali carb	Sharp, cutting pain, twitching of muscles Back or legs 'give out' Swellings Affinity to the knee and hip joints	< Cold weather < Lying on the painful side > Moving about

SCIATICA AND BRACHIAL NEURALGIA

When the muscles of the back become slack, the intervertebral joints and discs displace and this leads to pressure on the nerves. When the nerves affected are those that supply the leg the pain is referred down the leg and this is known as sciatica. Brachial Neuralgia is exactly the same pathological process as sciatica except that the nerves supply the arm(s). This table shows you some places to start with remedies for sciatica:

Remedy	Comments
Ammonium mur	< Sitting. Hamstrings feel short
Arsenicum album	Especially for older people
Colocynth	< Cold and damp
Dioscorea	> Extending the spine
Gelsemium	< Resting at night
Mag phos	Electric shooting pains down the leg

TENNIS ELBOW

This is a form of tendonitis at the exact point of the origin of the forearm abductor muscles. It is caused by overuse of the wrist in such activities as hammering, sewing and, er, tennis. Remedies to consider for Tennis & Golfer's Elbow include *Arnica, Bellis Perennis, Bryonia, Rhus Tox,* and *Ruta* – the "usual suspects".

GOLFER'S ELBOW

Is exactly the same as Tennis Elbow, except golfers have smaller balls…

CARPAL TUNNEL SYNDROME

Trauma, arthritis, myxoedema or oedema can damage the fibrous tissue which guides the flexor tendons through the carpal (anterior) tunnel, this damage leads to tingling and weakness of the fingers; a notable modality is that it is worse at night. Remedies to consider for Carpal Tunnel Syndrome include *Ruta, Calc Phos, Causticum* and *Hypericum.*

GOUT

Gout is caused by a build up of uric acid with which the kidneys can't cope. The uric acid crystallises in kidneys, cartilage or joint – typically in the toe. There may be genetic, dietary, or iatrogenic factors involved (iatrogenic describes a condition that has resulted from treatment of some form – often conventional medication – an unexpected disease state).

ANKYLOSING SPONDYLITIS

This is a disease that affects the cartilaginous joints, which are those that require less movement such as the spine and sternum. Ankylosing occurs when the joints calcify and then ossify (turn to bone). When there is no longer any movement available the joint is said to have ankylosed. As Spondylitis refers to the spine, Ankylosing Spondylitis refers specifically to this disease affecting the spine. Consequently stiffening of the spine is the main characteristic. The usual site where Ankylosing Spondylitis begins its manifestation is the sacro-iliac joint and this joint gets progressively stiffer in early to late middle age. AS however can be seen in other joints namely the hip joint, the shoulder girdle and even the soles of the feet. These sites, if affected, will be tender on palpation. Other complications of AS may include a general weakness, iritis and aortic damage. Remedies to consider for Ankylosing Spondylitis include *Aesculus, Kalmia Latifolia, Argentum Mur, Conium, Natrum Mur* and *Rhus Tox*.

REITERS SYNDROME

This consists of a triad of symptoms; namely conjunctivitis (or iritis), urethritis and arthritis. It generally follows an environmental trigger (most commonly Chlamydia – a parasite about the same size as a virus). Both Reiters syndrome and Ankylosing Spondylitis are forms of "reactive arthritis", the difference being that the trigger factors are not known for Ankylosing Spondylitis. Reiters Syndrome also affects large synovial joints as well as cartilage (Ankylosing Spondylitis only affects the cartilage joints).

PERTHES DISEASE

This disease is the result of trauma to the epiphysis of the bone during childhood. The epiphysis is the section of bone where the actual growth takes place and the hip, spine, wrist carpals and the metatarsals of the feet are particularly vulnerable. If, for example, the blood supply to any of those areas is restricted (by injury) the growing bone may soften for a while and may distort from pressure before growing again.

NERVE ENTRAPMENT SYNDROMES

This collection of disorders is caused by compression of nerves that run through places in the body that are unduly constricted. Naturally this can apply especially to the nerves running through the spine if there is any dislocation. Among the sort of diseases this can cause are (as previously mentioned) sciatica, carpal tunnel syndrome and brachial neuralgia. Symptoms include parasthaesia (pins and needles), shooting pains and weakness of the muscles, so the patient will drop things. The pains may be more marked on certain movements of the neck. A similar syndrome can affect the front of the thigh, known as meralgia parasthetica… further down the leg this sort of effect can be caused by sitting with one foot under the knee; causing foot drop.

GLOVE AND STOCKING DISTRIBUTION

This effect occurs in peripheral neuropathy where the damage to the nerves is caused by disease rather than mechanical damage. The neuropathy can be caused by toxins or drugs or can be secondary to established medical conditions such as alcoholism, vitamin deficiency allergy or diabetes mellitus (in which case the spread is slow and seen by gradual neuralgic pains and weakness).

These conditions can be loosely termed polyneuritis (if only one nerve is involved it is called mononeuritis). A particularly notorious type of polyneuritis can sometimes follow immunisation or acute viral infections such as herpes, measles or glandular fever. This is often referred to as Guillain Barre syndrome. The symptoms arrive rapidly (in hours) with tingling and numbness, which spread up the arms and legs hence glove and stocking syndrome. Recovery is usually complete and takes up to six months.

OSTEOPOROSIS

This is a loss of bony tissue resulting in bones that become brittle and liable to fracture. Causes include infection, injury and synovitis in a localised condition. Generalised osteoporosis is common in the elderly and in women following menopause and is one of the things that HRT is supposed to halt. The best remedies are probably good constitutional ones and appropriate tissues salt(s).

DIETARY CONSIDERATIONS

The problem of arthritis, gout and joint complaints is not a new one. Stone age skeletons show some signs of having problems with their joints. It is a fundamental verity that we were not designed to stand upright and consequently we are likely to suffer for it. It follows then that a dietary approach to joint disorders will not, in itself, be curative (in most cases) because the diet of our stone age ancestors was, on the whole, quite healthy. The reverse of the coin, however, is worth examining ... foods that exacerbate any conditions and those which may lead to musculo-skeletal problems. Joint problems, as they are acute inflammatory diseases, can sometimes result from an allergy reaction to certain foods or chemicals.

The foods that can have positive and beneficial effects are shown here. It's not much of a list and you wouldn't be too pleased to spend your life eating only this stuff; but if the alternative is RA it might be worth a go.

Category	Foods
The Absolutely Brilliant food . . . best of all.	Cabbage, celery, turnip, lemon, dandelion, oily fish.
Fruits	Cherries, strawberries, raspberries, pineapple, apple, plums, blackcurrants, gooseberries, melon, pears, grapes, banana, lemon.
Vegetables	Artichokes, carrots, cabbage, onion, leek, celery, chicory, olives, dandelions, jerusalem artichokes, fennel, radish, potatoes, turnips, nettles.
Grains	Rye, soya, brown rice, millet, buckwheat.
Nuts, Seeds and Pulses	Walnut, sprouted alfalfa, sprouted mung beans, beansprouts.
Herbs	Chervil, parsley, garlic, juniper, thyme, sage, chamomile, rosemary, marjoram.

SPINAL INJURY

If there's been an injury to the spine, you need to deal with the trauma. Go back to the blow and sort out what should have been done at the time of the trauma. We can see a range of symptoms that come from the blow thus: -

Example of symptoms arising from a blow to the spine	
Head pains Indigestion Weakness Blurred vision	Tiredness Stiffness Irritability Insomnia.

It may well be that none of these symptoms (if repertorised) would lead for example to *Arnica*. But *Arnica* may well be the remedy because of the aetiology of trauma. Major remedies to consider with such an aetiology are:

ARNICA

Arnica can overcome the obstacle of shock, no matter how distant in time; as Hahnemann would advocate, "overcome the obstacles to cure". The whole system has been shaken up and there's still an 'energy leak' (Murphy), so we prescribe to stop the leak. It is a prescription based on an energy level not a symptom level.

HYPERICUM

This remedy is indicated where there is evidence of a back trauma with nerve pain: sharp, shooting, numbness, tingling. Spinal concussion. Nerve paralysis. Sciatica. *Hypericum* can also prove beneficial post-childbirth; post-epidural and post-spinal tap.

NATRUM SULPHURICUM

A remedy that is good for stiffness, deep spinal ache < damp weather. Sometimes *Arnica* will only palliate, so use *Natrum Sulph*. The nearer you get to the neck, the more likely this remedy is to be indicated. Look for spinal trauma with personality change (e.g. depression related to pain). As an aside if the pain leads the patient to think of suicide, try *Aurum* or *Natrum sulph*. Often we treat depression etc. with *Ignatia, Natrum mur* and so on. But if the depression is due to a First Aid problem then cure that – fix the leak and the depression may well go away.

RUTA GRAVEOLENS

Ruta has been shown to be helpful in cases where there is a picture of back injury from torsion or twisting. Look for lameness and weakness in the back, any injuries from lifting or straining. The sensations are of a sharp shooting pain with a deep ache and, almost always, stiffness. *Ruta* also comes to mind where there is a slipped disc; especially since trauma. In my experience it's the number one remedy for over-manipulation from osteopathy or chiropractic. Patients can complain of a feeling of a knot or crick in the spine and frequently loss of flexibility. Consider *Ruta* for dislocation – not just in the spine, but also of the knee or shoulder.

The chronic of *Ruta* is *Calc fluor* (6c daily). You can use it acutely and then return to the *Ruta*. This is called periodic prescribing.

MAGNESIUM PHOSPHORICA

This is an acute 'back spasm' remedy; noted for sharp shooting pain which are > heat and also > pressure.

HEADACHES

There are many possible causes for headaches – musculoskeletal pathology being one, and consequently a number of chapters into which this small section could fit. However, as the musculoskeletal system is often the first area to look at when treating headaches, this seems to be an appropriate section to place them in.

Many headaches are classified as 'tension headaches'. Some sources suggest that as many as 85% fall into this category, making this an important area of musculoskeletal pathology.

You will have to treat many, many headaches, and they can be difficult. The Headache section of Murphy's Repertory is one of the largest and consequently a bit of a minefield to plough through. I would however, recommend that you at least read the section. It will give you a good idea of where to look when you are treating this incredibly common complaint.

The following table will, I hope, guide you towards some of the 'usual suspects' for tension headaches – those in which the pain is referred from the neck, shoulders, or back. The table deliberately focuses on headaches that have a muscular aetiology.

Remedy	Comments	Modalities
Bryonia	Headaches may be clearly associated with tension in the neck. Pain and dryness in the neck. Bursting, splitting headeache.	< motion > rest. Pain and swelling in the neck or back. < warmth, touch. > pressure, lying on painful side.
Gelsemium	Headache may be associated with dizziness, drowsiness, trembling and muscular weakness. Dull heavy headache.	Sore to touch. < damp weather, fog, before storm < bad news, smoking. > urinating, bending forward.
Phosphoric acid	Very debilitated by headache. Useful for adolescents. Heavy, crushing headache.	> keeping warm. < exertion. < from being talked to.
Picric acid	Headaches referred from the spine. Occipital head pains. Vertigo. Heavy, tired feeling.	> tight pressure. < mental exertion. > cold water.
Natrum mur	Coldness and emaciation in the neck. Throbbing, blinding headache – like hammers in the brain. Chronic headache with nausea.	< pre and post-menses. < sunrise to sunset. < noise, warmth, music. > open air, fasting, cold baths.
Calc phos	Headache at the 'top' of the head. School children's headaches. Headache with digestive disturbance.	< cold, damp weather. < melting snow. > in summer. > warm, dry atmosphere.
Silica	Headache clearly associated with back pain. Headache from not eating. Sweaty head –offensive	< in the morning. < washing, lying down, uncovering. > warmth, wrapping up. > wet, humid weather.
Lac caninum	Headache moves from side to side. Very weak-prostrated. Headache with blurred vision and/or nausea. Headache clearly associated with pain in the small of the back.	< in the morning of one day and the evening of the next. > cold cold drinks.
Graphites	Headaches with a 'rush of blood' to the head. Flushed face.Headache clearly associated with rheumatic pains on one side of the head-extending to the teeth.	< warmth, at night. <during and after menses. > in the dark. > wrapping up.

RED FLAGS

It is very important that you do not consider headaches in complete isolation. They can be pointers to other, sometimes vital, pathology. In absolute extreme cases a persistent headache can be an indication of brain tumour, so be thoughtful and pay particular attention to the possible source of the pain.

It's not uncommon for headaches have their 'root' in another pathology, or another area of the body (as in the table above). These are usually called 'referred' headaches; the pain is referred from one place to another. Typical examples would include headaches due to a muscular problem, or headaches caused by eyestrain. Other 'referred' headaches to look out for are:

VASCULAR HEADACHES

Where the underlying cause is to be found in the cardiovascular system – typically headaches due to high blood pressure

CONSTIPATION

Chronic constipation can lead to higher levels of toxins in the system than are healthy, and this is turn can lead to persistent headaches.

TENSION HEADACHES

These are due to a chronic contraction of muscles, examples include neck muscles, scalp and eye muscles, and tension during the day; usually > sleep.

MIGRAINE

Due to contraction then dilation of the blood vessels in the brain (and sometimes the visual cortex, hence the zigzag patterns, photophobia, and blurred vision). Aetiology can include stress, hormone change, diet and additives. There is also good evidence for a strong genetic link. Symptoms include: visual, tingling, neuralgia, red eyes and vomiting.

GLAUCOMA

Typified by a pain in the head, face and sometimes abdominal pain; all < night.

SINUSITIS

Check for tender sinuses, and of course, most patients who suffer with blocked sinuses will know that this is the cause of their headaches and hopefully will tell you.

TRIGEMINAL NEURALGIA

Patients will complain of sudden severe lancinating pain, < touch & chewing.

SUMMARY

There are, of course, any number of reasons why your patients may present with headaches. I would have two caveats for you when treating them; they're not always easy to cure, and also, as we've seen, there may be some underlying pathology. So, in this most common and simple ailment we may have to do our best work. There are no short cuts to dealing with headaches – take the case as fully as possible.

FURTHER READING

Ian Watson **A Guide to the Methodologies of Homœopathy**
Cutting Edge Publications
ISBN 0 9517657 0 1

Ian Watson **Aspects of Homœopathy – Musculo-Skeletal Problems**
Stramongrate Press
(No ISBN – Tel. 01922 – 685544)

Asa Hershoff **Homeopathy for Musculoskeletal Healing**
North Atlantic Books
ISBN 1-55643-237-2
www.amershamhealth.com

Dorothy Shepherd **The Magic of the Minimum Dose**
C W Daniel Company Ltd
ISBN 0852072988

Pulford **Repertory of the Symptoms of Rheumatism and Sciatica**
B Jain Publishers
ISBN 81-7021-112-3

NOTES

CONTENTS

THE NERVOUS SYSTEM

The nervous system, frankly, is a difficult area of anatomy & physiology to study. It is littered with possibilities for confusion and indecision regarding pathology. Most practitioners get plenty of patients who have diseases related to the nervous system, so it's an area where you need to try and establish some clarity.

The human nervous system is responsible for sending, receiving, and processing nerve impulses… as if you couldn't guess that. All of the body's muscles and organs rely upon these nerve impulses to function.

Three systems work together to carry out the mission of the nervous system: the central, the peripheral, and the autonomic nervous systems.

THE CENTRAL NERVOUS SYSTEM

Is responsible for issuing nerve impulses and analysing sensory data, and includes the brain and spinal cord.

THE PERIPHERAL NERVOUS SYSTEM

Carries nerve impulses to and from the body's many structures, and includes the many craniospinal nerves that branch off the brain and spinal cord.

THE AUTONOMIC NERVOUS SYSTEM

This comprises the sympathetic and parasympathetic systems and is responsible for regulating and coordinating the functions of vital structures in the body, such as heart rate, perspiration, salivation, and intestinal movements.

Definitions For This Page
Autonomic means involuntary. The Sympathetic Nervous System is the part of the autonomic nervous system which has an 'excitatory effect' – increasing blood flow to the limbs, opening airways in the lungs, etc. The Parasympathetic System has the opposite effect- a 'depressive effect', reducing heart rate etc.

The brain is the primary component of the nervous system, occupying the cranial cavity. Without its outermost protective membrane, the dura mater, the brain weighs an average of three pounds, comprising about 97% of the entire central nervous system. The brain is connected to the upper end of the spinal cord (which connects through the foramen magnum of the skull) and is responsible for issuing nerve impulses, processing nerve impulse data, and engaging in the higher order thought processes. The brain is divided into three parts: the large cerebrum, the smaller cerebellum, and the brainstem leading to the spinal cord. The brainstem is also descriptively divided into the medulla oblongata, the midbrain, and the pons.

In humans the brain is a mass of pinkish-grey tissue composed of about 100 billion nerve cells, each linked to another and together responsible for the control of all mental functions.

The brain, in addition to nerve cells (neurones), contains glial cells (supporting cells), blood vessels, and secretory organs. The brain is the control centre for movement, sleep, hunger, thirst, and virtually every other vital activity necessary to survival. All human emotions, including love, hate, fear, anger, elation, and sadness, are controlled by the brain. It also receives and interprets the countless signals that are sent to it from other parts of the body and from the external environment.

ANATOMY AND COMPOSITION

From the outside the brain appears as three distinct but connected parts: the cerebrum, the cerebellum, and the brain stem. The term brain stem usually refers to all the structures lying between the cerebrum and the spinal cord.

In addition, although the brain is well protected by the cranium, three membranes called meninges cover it. The outer one, the dura mater, is tough and shiny. The middle membrane, the arachnoid layer, encloses the brain loosely and does not slip down into the brain's convolutions, or ridges. The inner membrane, the pia mater, consists mainly of small blood vessels that adhere to the surface of the brain.

CEREBRUM

The cerebrum is the largest part of the human brain, making up approximately 85 percent of the brain's weight, its large surface area and intricate development account for the allegedly superior intelligence of humans, compared to other animals.

The cerebrum is divided by a longitudinal fissure into right and left, mirror-image hemispheres. The corpus callosum is the slab of white nerve fibres that connects these two cerebral hemispheres and transfers important information from one side of the brain to the other.

You may hear of disturbances to the pressure of the Cerebrospinal fluid (CSF). It is the CSF which circulates within these cerebral ventricles and around the spinal cord and serves to protect the inner part of the brain from varying pressures. It also transports chemical substances within the nervous system.

CEREBELLUM

The cerebellum lies in the posterior of the cranium, underneath the cerebral hemispheres. Like the cerebrum, it is made up of grey, unmyelinated cells on the exterior and white, myelinated cells in the interior. It is composed of two multi-ridged hemispheres that are connected by white fibres called the vermis.

The cerebellum is linked with the midbrain by the superior (top) peduncle, with the pons by the middle peduncle, and with the medulla by the inferior (bottom) peduncle. This is just for your information – what you really need to know is what it does, which is as follows…

The cerebellum is essential to the control of movement of the human body in space. It acts as a reflex centre for the coordination and precise maintenance of equilibrium. Voluntary muscle tone – as related to posture, balance, and equilibrium – is similarly controlled by this vital part of the brain. Thus, all motor activity, from hitting a cricket ball to fingering a violin, depends on the cerebellum.

BRAIN STEM

The brain stem is divided into several components, each of which is described below.

THALAMUS

This part of the forebrain consists of two rounded masses of grey tissue lying within the very middle of the brain, between the two hemispheres. It is the crucial relay station for incoming sensory signals and outgoing motor signals passing to and from the cerebral cortex. All sensory input to the brain, except that of the sense of smell, connects to individual nerve cells of the thalamus.

HYPOTHALAMUS

The hypothalamus lies just below the thalamus on the midline at the base of the brain. It is made up of distinct areas and nuclei. The hypothalamus regulates or is involved directly in the control of many of the body's vital activities and drives those that are necessary for survival: eating, drinking, temperature regulation, sleep, emotional behaviour and sexual activity.

MIDBRAIN

The mesencephalon is composed of three parts. The first consists of the cerebral peduncles, fibre systems that conduct impulses to and from the cerebrum. The second is the corpora quadrigemina, four bodies that relay signals through the visual and auditory pathways. The third is a central canal, called the aqueduct of Sylvius, around which is located grey matter that is important in pain and also possibly in addictive states.

Definitions for this page
Mesencephalon is another word for the midbrain.

PONS

Located between the medulla and midbrain, the pons is directly in front of the cerebellum. It consists mainly of transverse and longitudinal white nerve fibres that are interlaced in a complex network. A transverse bridge of fibres arises from the peduncles of the cerebellum and joins its two halves. An intricate longitudinal fibre system connects the medulla with the cerebral hemispheres. Located in the pons are a group of cells that act as relay stations and some of these are associated with the fifth, sixth, seventh, and eighth cranial nerves.

MEDULLA OBLONGATA

Situated between the spinal cord and pons, the medulla actually is a pyramid-shaped enlargement of the spinal cord. The origin of the reticular formation, an important network of nerve cells, makes up a large portion of this structure. The nuclei of origin of the 9th, 10th, 11th, and 12th cranial nerves also rest in the medulla. Impulses between the spinal cord and the brain are conducted through the medulla by means of ascending and descending fibre pathways. Within the medulla are the vital control centres for cardiac, vasoconstrictor, and respiratory functions, as well as other reflex activities, including vomiting. Damage to this structure usually results in immediate death.

CRANIAL NERVES

Twelve pairs of cranial nerves arise symmetrically from the base of the brain. They are distributed mainly to the structures of the head and neck and are numbered, from front to back, in the order in which they arise. Some are motor nerves, controlling muscle movement, others are sensory, and still others contain fibres for both sensory and motor impulses.

SUPPORTING VASCULAR SYSTEM

With all this activity going on, the brain needs a huge amount of blood. Necessary oxygen and glucose are supplied to brain cells by two sets of cranial arteries. Just below the neck, each of the common carotid arteries divides into an external branch, which carries blood to the outside of the cranium, and an internal branch, which supplies the forward portion of the brain. The remainder of the brain is supplied by the two vertebral arteries, which join together with the two internal carotid arteries to form the circle of Willis at the base of the brain. A whacking 25% of all the blood pumped by the heart is then circulated within the brain tissue by a large network of cerebral and cerebellar arteries.

FUNCTIONS OF THE CEREBRAL CORTEX

Physiologists and neurologists have spent a whole load of time and energy mapping areas of the cerebral cortex to localise and define the various regions. Noting, of course, those that are responsible for motor movement, sensory processes, memory and other cognitive functions. Early anatomical studies had already led to the naming of the various lobes, gyri (convolutions), and fissures.

THE PERIPHERAL NERVOUS SYSTEM

This refers to all parts of the nervous system that lie outside the Central Nervous System (ie. the brain and the spinal cord). As a system it includes the cranial nerves and the spinal nerves and their branches which link the receptors and effector organs with the brain and spinal cord. (Effector organs are the organs 'affected'...the organ or gland which has activity.) For our purposes let's start with the cranial nerves.

The Cranial nerves are numbered one to twelve and all have a name and a specific function. This is shown in the table below:

CRANIAL NERVES		
Number	**Name**	**Important Functions**
I	Olfactory	Smell
II	Optic	Sight
III	Oculomotor	Eyeball movement & regulation of the pupils
IV	Trochlear	Eyeball movements
V	Trigeminal	Movements of jaw, eardrum, ear bones, chewing
VI	Abducent	Eyeball movements
VII	Facial	Facial expression, secretions, taste
VIII	Auditory	Hearing and balance
IX	Glossopharyngeal	Movements of the pharynx, and larynx, taste
X	Vagus	Movements of the pharynx, and larynx, viscera, swallowing, secretions, controls respiration, slows heart
XI	Accessory	Movements of the head and shoulders
XII	Hypoglossal	Movements of the tongue

THE ANATOMY OF NERVES

The building block of the nervous system is the neurone (or nerve cell), which has a cell body around a central nucleus.

The dendrites are the shorter branches of the cell body of the neurone. These make contact with other neurones at synapses and then carry nerve impulses into the cell body.

The longer process which extends from the nerve centre is the nerve fibre, the axon. The axon extends away from the body of the neurone and carries nerve impulses away from it. An axon may be over a metre in length (in certain neurones). In large nerves the axon has a sheath called the neurilemma made of myelin which is interrupted at intervals by gaps called the nodes of Ranvier, at which branches of the axon may leave. The axon ends by dividing into several branches called the telodendria, which make contact with other nerves or with muscle or gland membranes. Neurones with myelin sheaths are called myelinated (go on!) and without the sheath, you guessed it, they're called non-myelinated. The function of the myelin sheath is to:

- Increase the speed of the nerve impulse
- Insulate the nerve
- Protect the nerve

These cell bodies tend to make up the "grey matter" of the nervous system while the "white matter" is the myelin. A myelin sheath is really a cell – a Schwann Cell which 'wraps itself' around the axon – up to 20 times.

I'm not going to go into detail on the electro-chemical changes involved in the nerve impulses, save to say that Sodium, Potassium and Chlorine are the chemicals involved (which may sometimes be pertinent to homœopaths when choosing a remedy) and that the process of electrical change is done "in chunks" in the myelinated nerves thereby speeding the action of the impulse.

The dendrites, then, connect to other neurones and the space between the synaptic end bulb of one neurone and the dendrites of another neurone is called the Synapse and it is across this gap that chemical transmitters cause the next cell body to stimulate 'action potential'.

If the synaptic end bulbs conclude with muscle fibres we call them Muscle End Plates, this sort of neurone (ie. one which affects movement) is called a Motor nerve neurone.

Sensory nerves, obviously, form the start of the feedback process by which the brain receives information. They differ primarily from motor neurons in the direction of the information and action flow.

THE AUTONOMIC NERVOUS SYSTEM

Among the motor fibres may be found groups that carry impulses to viscera. (Viscera, my dears, means the organs within the body cavities.) These fibres are designated by the special name of autonomic nervous system. That system consists of two divisions, more or less antagonistic in function, that emerge from the central nervous system at different points of origin.

One division, the sympathetic, arises from the middle portion of the spinal cord, joins the sympathetic ganglionated chain, courses through the spinal nerves, and is widely distributed throughout the body.

The other division, the parasympathetic, arises both above and below the sympathetic, that is, from the brain and from the lower part of the spinal cord. These two divisions control the functions of the respiratory, circulatory, digestive, and urogenital systems.

The autonomic nervous system is responsible for the self-controlling aspects of the body's nervous network, and is under the control of the cerebral cortex, the hypothalamus, and the medulla oblongata. Working in tandem with the central nervous system, the autonomic nervous system features two sub-systems which regulate body functions such as involuntary smooth muscle movement and heart rate.

The two sub-systems are known as the sympathetic and parasympathetic nervous systems, and their functions, as noted above, operate in opposition to one another, delicately balancing the bodily functions that they control.

THE SYMPATHETIC NERVOUS SYSTEM

The sympathetic nervous system causes fight or flight responses in moments of stress or stimulus, such as increased heart rate, saliva flow, and perspiration.

THE PARASYMPATHETIC NERVOUS SYSTEM

The parasympathetic system counterbalances these effects by slowing the heart rate, dilating blood vessels, and relaxing involuntary smooth muscle fibres.

PERIPHERAL NEUROPATHY

Neuropathy is any disease that affects the peripheral nerves, so peripheral neuropathy is a bit tautologous. Nonetheless it is the name given to a bunch of diseases and we need to look at them briefly, for reasons that will become apparent.

The peripheral nerves are liable to disease arising from interference to the blood vessels that supply them, or from direct poisoning from drugs or toxins or, indeed from allergic reaction. In a clinical setting you will most often see neuropathy as a secondary symptom to an established disease (diabetes, alcoholism, vitamin deficiency, etc.). The symptoms will be described as weakness and/or numbness. Sometimes the 'pins and needles' description will apply. In mononeuropathy a single nerve is affected and in polyneuropathy several (or even all) peripheral nerves are affected.

GUILLIAN BARRE SYNDROME

One form of polyneuritis is the Guillain Barre Syndrome. This can follow immunisation or acute viral infections like glandular fever, mumps, and herpes. The neuropathy arrives a couple of weeks after the initial infection (or vaccination) and the symptoms arrive suddenly within a space of a few hours. The tingling starts in the feet and hands, leading to the 'glove and stocking symptom'. The disease then spreads up towards the trunk. It may be so global that the patient needs to be put on a respirator, but they usually retain consciousness. Recovery time can be six months or more.

BELL'S PALSY

This is a condition of the seventh cranial nerve (which as you no doubt recall is the one which supplies the muscles of facial expression and taste). It is a disease that paralyses one side of the face. A person who has Bell's palsy cannot wrinkle the forehead or close the eye on the affected half of the face. The mouth sags on one side. With effort, the victim can move the facial muscles on the healthy side, but the face is distorted because the muscles on the other side cannot be moved.

The symptoms of Bell's palsy appear suddenly in most cases. Some pain may be felt for one or two days before they occur, but the paralysis itself is painless. Most of those afflicted lose the sense of taste on one side of the tongue. The eye on the paralysed side becomes dry. Sounds may seem extremely loud at times.

Bell's palsy is caused by a sudden swelling of the main motor nerve on one side of the face. A bony canal surrounds this nerve, and the nerve runs through it at a point where it exits the middle ear. Typically the nerve will swell if exposed to cold draughts for a long time. The swollen nerve presses against the canal, causing the nerve to function improperly. A virus may also cause the swelling of the nerve.

More than 90% of the of Bell's palsy sufferers recover in several weeks, even without treatment. But in some cases, the symptoms become permanent. In its early stages, Bell's palsy can often be treated with steroid drugs. For those of us still convinced that homœopathy could do better, the remedies to look at are *Belladonna, Causticum, Aconite,* and *Gelsemium.*

If that really doesn't cover it, look under Face, paralysis, Murphy, page 593.

MYALGIC ENCEPHALOMYELITIS (ME)

This largely unpronounceable disease is (if my experience is anything to go by) one which will drift into your practice quite regularly and may occupy more than its fair share of your time.

The foremost symptoms are pain and fatigue and the affected population (at the start of the disease) are those aged between 10 and 30. It has been my experience that there is a familial connection, but I haven't seen this in the literature.

SIGNS AND SYMPTOMS

Muscular pain and stiffness, swollen glands, headache, numbness, muscle twitching, sore throat, depression, panic attacks, and sometimes fever, dyspnoea and diarrhoea. As the disease moves to a more chronic state the residue may be muscle fatigue, exhaustion and insomnia.

Medical research into ME has moved in two different directions and come up with two options as to cause…… metabolic and viral. Because the pancreas is important in the maintenance of glucose (and therefore energy) in the body and because some ME sufferers are found to be hypoglycaemic periodically and to develop symptoms after their meals, it is thought that this organ may be damaged in some way. Pancreas organ remedies include *Senna, Iris Versicolor, Natrum Sulph* and *Phosphorus* – all at about 3x to 6x potency.

It is also widely believed to be established that the initial stages of the disease are the result of a virus, the Coxsackie virus or the polio virus – because antibodies of these viri can be seen in the blood. Certainly post-viral fatigue is not uncommon and ME may be a particularly extended version of this.

CONVENTIONAL TREATMENT

There is generally little effective conventional treatment available. In general ME sufferers are left to their own devices; this often leads to an interest in alternative therapies, hence the arrival of these patients at your clinic.

HOMŒOPATHIC TREATMENT

This is one of those conditions where homœopathy can be of enormous help. Sadly there are no short cuts. It really does pay to attend closely to the presenting symptoms and address the case on the immediate presentation and follow up (or coincide) with well-chosen constitutional remedies.

INSOMNIA

This is one of the more popular nervous system disorders; we'll see it as the main presenting complaint or a concomitant in about a third of all cases, so it's well worth getting good at treating it. There are many, many causes of insomnia so it's vitally important when treating it to find the cause of the problem. Very often we'll take a case and arrange the presenting symptoms into a hierarchy (often using Kent or some other luminary to give our symptoms some 'order') and then repertorise the case. However, insomnia is one of a number of pathologies that may not yield itself to this sort of approach. What's important therefore is understanding the focus of the case.

Robin Murphy cites an example in one of his taped lectures, where a woman suffers from very heavy periods, which lead to a loss of blood, this in turn leads her to become weak and irritable to her loved ones. Her irritability leads to arguments and the ruminative thoughts of these arguments go round and round in her head during the night. Perhaps she feels guilty or angry or both. All this causes her to lose sleep. In a case like this, we as homœopaths, as 'practical prescribers' should be dealing with the heavy periods. It is her extensive haemorrhaging that is the ultimate cause of her insomnia, and no amount of repertorising such symptoms as irritability, guilty feelings, anger towards loved ones, and so forth, will help with the insomnia. It is most important to address the central weakness, the sensitivity of the system. When that is done, the insomnia will fade away.

Robin has a wonderful word for these symptoms; he calls them "floaters". Not a word that translates all that well across the Atlantic, it has to be said, but nonetheless it's a fantastically useful concept. In this instance the floaters are symptoms that form a 'pathway' to the presenting complaint . . . this causes that, and that causes something else, and that causes insomnia. Of course it is perfectly possible to have floaters going in the other direction (i.e. leading away from the presenting complaint). Insomnia causes tiredness, this makes the patient tearful, sensitive to noise, unable to do their job, which leads to worries about position and money, and so forth.

In either example it's important to focus on the central disturbance in the case, and to deal with that. What we're trying to do is to centre our thoughts on the evolution of the symptoms, often the chronology of the case. In the heavy bleeding to insomnia case it is relatively easy to see. The important lesson from cases like these is that imposing a pre-ordained hierarchy of symptoms (e.g. the Kentian hierarchy) will not always lead us to a well-chosen remedy. It may do sometimes, but that can be as much a matter of luck as anything else, so beware of trying to shoehorn every case into a system – sometimes it just won't work.

Insomnia is a classic example of this type of case (although it could be argued that there are very many others). The causation of the case may be physical (heavy periods), mental (high pressure occupation), or emotional (a recent bereavement). Any change up or down in any of these factors can lead to insomnia. Additionally, we need to look at other exacerbating factors, including drug effects, alcohol abuse, environmental issues, and so on.

When you're taking an insomnia case then, try and be sure about the thing that's 'exciting' the patient, and go there first for your remedies. In my experience if you ask a patient why they can't sleep they most often reply that they don't know . . . "I just can't sleep". It's hardly surprising really; our culture isn't really geared towards looking for a deeper reason. So try and find out what they're doing whilst they're awake. If pressed most people will tell you priceless information about the case. Someone will say that they are lying awake and they're thinking about the work they did the previous day, and what they've got to do tomorrow, and the annual budget and . . . well you get the picture. This is the sort of information we need; if we look up 'Insomnia' in Murphy's Repertory we find nearly 20 columns of rubrics, so we need to get a bit more specific with our cases. Sometimes the insomnia can be linked clearly to a physical problem, if we ask what the patient is doing whilst awake, they may say "Oh I have to go to the toilet" or "I'm just really achy" or "the slightest noise wakes me". Often these responses will steer us towards an appropriate remedy or set of rubrics.

So . . . let's look at some of the 'usual suspects' for treating insomnia:

CALCAREA CARBONICA

This is a good remedy for children who can't sleep. Something most of our mothers said at one time or another is that we'll sleep better if we have a glass of milk before bed. These kinds of 'old wives tales' have carried so far down the years because they have a big chunk of truth in them. The calcium in the milk actually does aid sleep.

This is one of the first remedies to think of for children who have nightmares, especially if the nightmares are of monsters. This is the sort of case where the child has been watching one of the big movies of the year – recently the 'Harry Potter' or 'Lord of the Rings' series – and when they sleep they dream of monsters which makes them afraid to fall back to sleep. Actually some of the big blockbuster movies of the last decade or so have been pretty scary (think of the 'Jurassic Park' series) but they are squarely aimed at the young market. I have found that *Calcarea carbonica* will really help these children. Potency doesn't seem to be an issue with this remedy, I've found 200c in one dose or 6c daily to be equally effective.

. . . as an aside
If you are treating a child who suffers from nightmares, bad dreams, and is generally 'scared of the dark' and who becomes whiny and weepy insisting on coming into the parent's bedroom and sleeping with mum and dad, they will often need Pulsatilla. Children who suffer from poor sleep due to indigestion also benefit from Pulsatilla.

Adults who need *Calcarea carbonica* are the sort of people who suffer from ruminative thoughts. (Ruminating is what cows do with their food – they chew it over and over, this is a beautifully descriptive word when applied to psychology, people chew over and over their thoughts. We've all had some experience of this process, most commonly after an argument when one goes away from the fight and starts to play it over again in the memory thinking "... if I'd only said that, and he would have said this, and I could have said that" and so on.) So the adult *Calcarea carbonica* is a ruminator; they have worrying, persistent and tormenting thoughts. A few doses of *Calcarea carbonica* can really help.

AURUM METALLICUM

This is a good remedy for severe insomnia. I've found it to be particularly useful for elderly patients. It is a remedy associated with depression and the time when it is most common for a patient to feel worthless, useless, and despondent, and that there's no point in life anymore is just after retirement. This is a good remedy for 'the great retired'. The other life event which engenders these feeling (and consequently the *Aurum metallicum* state) is a devastating medical diagnosis – cancer being the most frequent.

The causative factors in *Aurum metallicum* are pain, depression and fear. So in addition to patients with an emotional aetiology this is good for those for whom pain is behind their insomnia.

KALI PHOSPHORICUM

This is bound to be helpful in insomnia as it is a great 'nerve tonic'. The typical picture is of someone who has insomnia whose genesis lies in his or her work. They are people who use their mind at work, and they may have been working too hard – insomnia from mental work. They come back from the office after a busy day and they can't switch off. Everything is still buzzing round in their head. For them the insomnia is a double blow because they are exhausted and still they can't sleep because their mind just won't slow down.

KALI CARBONICUM

If you look this remedy up and read around it, the literature says that they suffer from insomnia from 2 a.m. to 4 a.m. To be frank, I've found that a lot of time aggravations are less than helpful. For a start patients are often a little vague about these times, and they quite rightly say that not every night is the same. Also, if we allow an hour or so either side of the stated aggravation time we've pretty well covered the whole time that insomnia is a real problem! Nonetheless, that's what the books say about the Kali carbonicum time aggravation, so it may be useful to you.

This is a remedy that has physical concomitants with the insomnia. They can suffer from asthma – commonly saying that wheezing at night is a problem. One of the key features of the *Kali carbonicum* asthma is that they have a cold chest. The remedy also has heart troubles with palpitations being a characteristic. Oddly, in heart conditions there is a burning sensation as opposed to the cold chest typical of the asthma. In my experience this has been a very helpful remedy, when indicated, for patients who suffer from backache. Backache is a common cause of insomnia and as the Kali carbonicum patient is hypersensitive to pain, you can expect this remedy to provide some much-needed relief.

COFFEA CRUDA

This is a remedy that tests the faith of your patients – they can't sleep and you are proposing to give them some coffee! However, it is an excellent acute remedy for sleeplessness. Particularly it can help if the insomnia is arising from anticipation of a big event. I've found it to be great for children (and the young at heart) who are getting excited about Christmas, or birthday parties, an impending holiday, or a performance of some kind.

. . . as an aside
Coffea cruda is a great remedy for anticipation of pleasant events. Argentum nitricum is a good remedy for anticipation of unpleasant events. . . . and Gelsemium for anticipation of painful events.

IGNATIA

This is another remedy that has ruminative thoughts, going over conversations that they had during the day, especially if the conversations had some emotional impact. As one of the great homœopathic grief remedies it's an obvious candidate for insomnia following grief, but actually it's very useful for insomnia following any emotional trauma. One other causation that is typical of *Ignatia* is indecision. If they are lying awake at night unable to choose where to go on holiday, which car to buy, what career to opt for, and so on, *Ignatia* may help them to clarify their thoughts and finally settle down for a good night's sleep.

SULPHUR

This is one of the huge remedies in the homœopathic literature and so is bound to be of use in insomnia. The most likely cause of their sleep loss is likely to be intellectual ruminating. They spend the night thinking of great schemes, 'get-rich-quick' schemes, or the intellectual thoughts of the day carry over into the night. They just can't switch their brain off if they have an exciting idea...and of course *Sulphur* patients have a lot of exciting ideas. Oh, and don't forget they'll be too hot in bed!

THE HOMŒOPATHIC SLEEPING PILL

I have found the combination of *Ferrum phosphoricum, Kali phosphoricum,* and *Magnesia phosphorica* to be pretty useful as an acute remedy that can be taken as required by patients who are having difficulty adjusting their sleep patterns.

I generally use it in 6c potency, and have prescribed it with good results for shift workers especially those who do some day shifts, then some nights, then back to days and also for pilots and cabin crew coming back from long-haul flights. I usually suggest that the patient keeps a bottle next to the bed, and then they have one tablet before sleep and one if they wake up.

One airline captain said this was the most useful thing he'd ever been given in twenty years of flying. I was about to assume a suitably modest expression when he said that the bottle was exactly the right size to prop open his bedroom window for the perfect amount of fresh air. Homœopathy works in mysterious ways!

THE BRAIN

STROKES

This term derives from the Greek, and the old fashioned name is Apoplexy (to be "struck down"), this is how you may well see strokes described in the homœopathic literature.

A stroke is damage to the brain due to a blockage in blood flow, or to a haemorrhage of blood vessels in the brain. Without blood supply, sections of brain tissue quickly deteriorate or die, resulting in paralysis of the limbs or organs controlled by the affected brain area. Most strokes are associated with high blood pressure or arteriosclerosis, or both.

SIGNS & SYMPTOMS

Some of the signs of major stroke are facial weakness, inability to talk, loss of bladder control, difficulty in breathing and swallowing, and paralysis or weakness, particularly on one side of the body.

In the medical literature we often see strokes referred to as cerebral apoplexy or cerebrovascular accident (CVA). Strokes are the third commonest cause of death in over 65's (after coronary heart disease and cancer) affecting about one in 500 people. The good news for your patients is that one in three who have a stroke will completely recover in time. The majority of stroke cases are due to arterial blockage caused by either thrombosis or embolism.

THROMBOSIS

Thrombosis involves the gradual building up of fatty substances, or arteriosclerotic plaque, in one or more of the four arteries leading to the brain. As these arteries become narrowed, a potential stroke victim often experiences recurrent warnings of transient paralysis, maybe in one arm or leg or on one side of the face. They may also discover impairments in speech, vision, or other motor functions. At this stage, deposits in the linings of the cerebral arteries can often be treated by surgery, including laser surgery and microsurgical bypass of blockages. Anticoagulant drugs, changes in diet, and even daily doses of aspirin are also used. Actual thrombosis occurs when an artery has occluded (become blocked), leading to permanent brain damage.

EMBOLISM

Embolism occurs when a cerebral artery suddenly becomes blocked by material coming from another part of the bloodstream. Such solid masses are called emboli, and often form as clots in a diseased or malfunctioning heart, but can also come from dislodged fragments of arteriosclerotic plaque or even an air bubble. If the embolism is small it may be broken up quite quickly by the flow of blood, thus the symptoms are only transient. These episodes are referred to as Transient Ischaemic Attacks (TIA's). Treatment is largely preventive, consisting of monitoring of the diet, and, if possible, use of anticoagulants.

Definitions for this page
Arteriosclerosis refers to a condition that affects the arteries – either through calcium deposits in the arteries or thickening of the walls of small arteries.

HAEMORRHAGE

Haemorrhaging of cerebral blood vessels is a less frequent cause of stroke and occurs most often where aneurysms, or blister-like bulges, develop on the forks of large cerebral arteries on the brain surface. The rupture of aneurysms causes brain damage, due to either the seeping of blood into brain tissue or the reduced flow of blood to the brain beyond the point of rupture.

HOMŒOPATHIC TREATMENT

As it is extremely unlikely that treatment will be available whilst a patient is actually having a stroke, the remedy emphasis is on post-stroke care. Remedies to consider particularly to help patients post-stroke are *Arnica* and *Kali mur* from 6x to 200c potency; these remedies have been shown to be useful in combination for patients in their recovery phase. As usual though there are plenty of remedies to choose from. (This is a common disease don't forget), so here is a table showing the major stroke remedies:

Remedy	Comments	Modalities
Aconite	Characterised by suddenness and fear. Great anxiety and fear of death. Numb and tingling extremities.	> open air. < warm room.
Anacardium	Impairment of memory – absent mindedness. May swear.	> eating.
Arnica	Number one stroke remedy. Red face. Sore, lame, bruised feeling (as usual).	< touch. > lying down.
Bartya carb	Loss of confidence. Bashful. Aversion to strangers. Senility. Child-like.	< washing. > open air.
Belladonna	Hot, red, throbbing. Violent, sudden onset. Delirium, furious, acuity of senses.	< touch, jar. > bending backwards.
Cocculus	Spasmodic affections which affect one half of the body. Feels hollow. Time passes quickly. Sadness.	< touch, noise, jar.
Gelsemium	Motor paralysis, dizzy, drowsy, droopy, dull and trembling. Apathy regarding the illness.	< bad news. > urination.
Hydrocyanicum Acidium	Convulsions and paralysis. Collapse. Hysterical convulsions.	Fears everything.
Ipecacuanha	Persistent nausea and vomiting. Irritable.	

Continued overleaf...

Remedy	Comments	Modalities
Lachesis	Talkative, restless, suspicious.	< after sleep > discharges.
Nux vomica	Irritable ++, sullen. Time passes too slowly.	< morning. > evening.
Opium	Depression, stupor, painlessness. Sleepy, sweaty, delirious.	< heat. > cold.

CEREBRAL INJURY

After a blow to the head, a person may be stunned or in a daze or may become unconscious for a moment. This injury, called a concussion, usually leaves no permanent damage. If the blow is more severe, causing haemorrhage and swelling, then severe headache, dizziness, paralysis, a convulsion, or temporary blindness may result, depending on the area of the brain affected. Choose *Arnica* immediately, and consider *Natrum Sulph* if there is an aetiology of a blow to the head.

MENINGITIS

This is an inflammatory condition of the meninges or membranes covering the brain and spinal cord. The inflammation is caused by a virus or bacteria (specifically the bacteria responsible for pneumonia, syphilis or tuberculosis).

SIGNS AND SYMPTOMS

The standard symptoms of Meningitis are: intense headache, fever, loss of appetite, intolerance to light and sound and rigidity of muscles in the neck. Sometimes there can be rigidity of the muscles of the leg (particularly the hamstring) – this is called Kernig's sign. In severe cases of meningitis we can see vomiting, convulsions, and delirium; leading eventually to death.

CONVENTIONAL TREATMENT

BACTERIAL AND VIRAL MENINGITIS

Bacterial meningitis is treated with antibiotics or sulphonamides. Viral meningitis does not respond to drugs. The traditional response is prolonged bed rest, darkness and quiet.

Viral meningitis is a non-fatal form of meningitis. Almost always affecting children, the disease produces symptoms of headache, high fever, vomiting, and leg pains. Patients with most types of viral meningitis usually recover spontaneously within one or two weeks.

Most cases of meningitis, particularly those caused by bacteria, have an abrupt onset, with symptoms including headache, stiff neck, fever, nausea, vomiting, listlessness, and irritability, sometimes leading to stupor and coma. It progresses rapidly and may lead to death if untreated in 24 to 72 hours.

Bacterial meningitis is usually very effectively treated by early administration of antibiotics. It's important for complementary therapists to be aware of this. This is one of the times when it may be appropriate to allow concerned parents to follow the conventional option and then deal with any ill effects from the antibiotics afterwards. If there is an outbreak of meningitis in the area (usually the local school) then *Belladonna* 12x daily (or 30c SSD) may be used as a prophylactic remedy. *Belladonna* may also be the remedy of choice in the early stages… up to 10M.

Occasionally, particularly in small children who are not treated early, serious brain damage may result. This may occur when drainage of spinal fluid from the cavities inside the brain is blocked, causing distension of the cavities, pressure on the brain, and enlargement of the skull, a condition that is called hydrocephalus. Consequently, swift conventional treatment may be the preferable option.

HOMŒOPATHIC TREATMENT

There is no reason why homœopathy cannot deal very successfully with meningitis. I would, however, caution you to be very sure that the child gets checked out by their doctor as soon as possible. It does no harm to give the remedy and then send them to see the Doctor. The remedies to consider are shown in this table, below:

Remedy	Comments
Belladonna	The number one remedy. Convulsions, pain, hot, red skin. Flushed face, staring eyes, etc.
Aconite	Sudden onset. Acute and violent attack. Tingling cold and numb. Children's Rx. < night.
Phosphorous	Chronic meningitis. Heat rising from the spine.
Helleborus	Complete unconsciousness. Rolls head. Sinking sensation.
Stramonium	Endless chatter. Desires light and company. Raises head from the pillow.
Zinc	Convulsions with a pale face and no heat. Very sensitive to noise. Child repeats everything.
Apis	Oedema. Red rosy hue, stinging pains, intolerance of heat and touch.

EPILEPSY

This is a chronic brain disorder characterised by repeated convulsions or seizures resulting from underlying brain damage, as opposed to those caused by hypoglycaemia or adverse drug reactions.

Epileptic seizures differ with the type of condition and may consist of loss of consciousness, convulsive jerking of parts of the body, emotional explosions, or periods of mental confusion. Studies show that although epilepsy is not inherited, predisposition to the disorder is a hereditary trait.

In persons suffering from epilepsy, the brain waves, which are manifestations of electrical activity in the cerebral cortex have a characteristically abnormal rhythm produced by excessive and simultaneous nerve-cell discharges. Furthermore, the wave patterns differ markedly according to type. Recordings of the brain waves are therefore important in the diagnosis and study of the disease and are obtained by means of a device called the electroencephalograph (ECG).

CONVENTIONAL TREATMENT

No specific cure for epilepsy exists, but seizures can be prevented or reduced in frequency in nearly 90 percent of the patients by the administration of drugs. Commonly anti-convulsant drugs are used. These have two functions; firstly to reduce the risk of a fit, and secondly to stop one that is in progress.

In the majority of cases you'll see in clinic, the drugs will be prophylactic. Consequently you have to be very careful about reducing or stopping them. An added complication can arise for epileptics in that some of them are only allowed to drive (operate machinery, etc.) if they have been 'fit-free' for a year or two. If you stop their drugs, even one fit can cost them dear. There can also be a risk of brain damage from continued fits and so cessation is important.

The anticonvulsant drugs have an inhibitory effect on brain activity, this means that they reduce the excessive electrical activity that both characterises and causes the fit. Naturally this inhibitory effect cannot be specific (ie. it is global in its operation), which can cause impairment to memory, concentration, coordination and energy. This is one of the areas in which conventional pharmacy agrees with homœopathy that the dose needs to be individualised. Generally patients are given a small dose, gradually increasing until the therapeutic effect outweighs the 'side effects'. In many cases the side effects are transitory anyway. Apart from these side effects there is also a serious risk of rebound effect if the drugs are stopped or if, for any reason the therapeutic dose is not maintained; which will almost certainly result in a fit.

The anticonvulsant drugs used include Diazepam, Carbamazepine, Clobazam, Phenobarbitone and Sodium Valproate. In a prolonged fit the drug of choice will often be intravenous valium (diazepam) which can stop the fit.

The most common drug used, in my experience, is Carbamazepine (Tegrotol). Here are some of its side effects: nausea & vomiting, dizziness, drowsiness, headache, ataxia (shaky movement and unsteady gait), confusion and agitation (elderly), visual disturbances (especially double vision), constipation, diarrhoea, anorexia, rashes (very common), leucopenia (reduction in the number of white blood cells), other blood disorders including thrombocytopenia (reduction in the number of platelets in the blood which leads to bleeding into the skin and/or spontaneous bleeding), agranulocytosis (low white cell production), and aplastic anaemia. Other side effects (yes there's more) include cholestatic jaundice (essentially obstructive jaundice – due to failure of normal amounts of bile to reach the intestines), hepatitis, acute renal failure and Stevens – Johnson Syndrome. Stevens-Johnson syndrome is a severe form of Erythema Multiforme (abnormal flushing of the skin) characterized by blistery lesions on the mucous membranes of the mouth, throat, ano-genital region, eyelids and corneal lining (conjunctiva).

HERE ARE YET MORE OF THE SIDE EFFECTS OF CARBAMAZEPINE:

Toxic epidermal necrolysis (dead skin to you and me), alopecia (baldness), thromboembolism (where a blot clot formed at one point in the circulation moves and becomes lodged at another point – which brings us back to strokes, which is where we came in). Other side effects include arthralgia (painful swelling of the joint), fever, proteinuria, lymph node enlargement, cardiac arrhythmia, dyskinesia (involuntary movements), paraesthesia (pins and needles), depression (what a surprise), impotence, gynaecomastia (men with boobs), galactorrhoea (copious or unexpected milk production), aggression, psychosis (if latent), photosensitivity, pulmonary hypersensitivity with dyspnoea and/or pneumonitis (inflammation of the alveoli), hyponatraemia (the presence in the blood of very low traces of sodium – usually associated with dehydration) and oedema.

Lovely! The point of this degree of painstaking detail is to remind you that you need to do your research. You need to know when you are treating someone exactly what their medication is doing (carbamazepine is not an uncommon medication), so that you can be sure whether you're treating a disease or a side effect. And so that your patient knows too.

Because epileptic seizures vary in intensity and in symptoms, epilepsy is divided into the following three major types: grand mal, petit mal, and psychomotor.

GRAND-MAL EPILEPSY

The onset of an attack of grand-mal epilepsy is often signaled by an involuntary scream, caused by contraction of the respiratory muscles. As loss of consciousness sets in, the entire body is gripped by a spastic muscular contraction. The face becomes red, the breathing is arrested, and the back arched. Subsequently, alternate contractions and relaxations of the muscles throw the body into such violent agitation that the patient is subject to serious injury. A folded handkerchief in the mouth may help prevent tongue and cheeks from being bitten during a seizure. After the convulsion subsides, the patient is exhausted and may sleep heavily. Fatigue and depression are often experienced upon awakening, and occasionally the patient has no memory of the seizure. Attacks occur at varying intervals, in some cases as seldom as once a year and in others as frequently as several times a day.

Seizures may occur successively with no intervening period of consciousness; this condition, known as status epilepticus, affects approximately 8% of those subject to grand-mal attacks and may be fatal unless treated promptly with diazepam or other drugs.

PETIT-MAL EPILEPSY

In petit-mal epilepsy the seizures are characterised by a sudden, momentary loss or impairment of consciousness. Overt symptoms are often as slight as an upward staring of the eyes, a staggering gait, or a twitching of the facial muscles. The patient often carries on without realising that the seizure has occurred.

PSYCHOMOTOR EPILEPSY

In psychomotor epilepsy the main symptom is amnesia. Duration of the seizures varies from a few minutes to several hours. Activity of the patient does not cease during the seizure, although behaviour may be totally unrelated to the environment. Also called temporal-lobe epilepsy, this form of seizure can be preceded by an aura (abdominal discomfort, dizziness, or strange odours and sensations). Some severe forms of temporal-lobe epilepsy are successfully treated by surgical removal of the damaged part of the brain.

HOMŒOPATHIC TREATMENT

There are plenty of remedies to choose from as far as epilepsy is concerned. Certainly you should be thinking of the 'brain goes off bang' remedies such as *Belladonna* and *Hyoscyamus*, but Murphy (Diseases page 407) offers a huge rubric of opportunity. Here are also a few hints courtesy of Clarke, from his 'Prescriber':

Acute Epilepsy		
Remedy	**Comments**	**Clarke's Potency**
Kali cyanatum	Falls insensible, turns blue, violent convulsions, dyspnoea.	3x
Belladonna	Recent attack in young sanguine subjects (sanguine – 'having the colour of blood' i.e. a ruddy, florid complexion, plethoric.)	1x – 3x
Kali bromatum	Epilepsy with mental hebetude (hebetude means stupidity) at each period.	30c
Absinthium	Petit mal epilepsy.	3x
Cicuta virosa	Violent convulsions, frightful distortions of eyes and limbs, opisthotonus.	3x

Chronic Epilepsy		
Remedy	**Comments**	**Clarke's Potency**
Bufo	Chronic epilepsy in general.	6c
Calc carb	In pale lymphatic subjects.	6c
Silica	Fits occur during sleep. Nervous irritability.	6c
Opium	Fits in sleep, drowsiness, constipation.	3x
Plumbum	Very obstinate constipation, cachexia, (abnormally low weight) malnutrition, unhealthy skin.	30c

MULTIPLE SCLEROSIS

This is a chronic disorder of the central nervous system (CNS) that causes the destruction of the covering (myelin sheath) over the nerves. The course of this disease is variable; it may advance, relapse, remit, or stabilise. The demyelinating plaques or patches are scattered throughout the central nervous system and interfere with the ability of the nerves to communicate (neurotransmission) causing a wide range of neurological symptoms.

SIGNS & SYMPTOMS

The symptoms of Multiple Sclerosis can vary greatly. Some people may have visual impairment (including blind spots), double vision (diplopia), or involuntary rhythmic movements of the eyes (nystagmus). People with Multiple Sclerosis may also experience impairment of speech, numbness or tingling sensation in the limbs and difficulty walking.

Dysfunction of the bladder and bowel may also be present. Multiple Sclerosis is rarely fatal; the average life expectancy is 93% of that of the general population. One in 5 Multiple Sclerosis patients experience one attack, followed by little or no advance in the disorder. Two-thirds of patients can walk independently 25 years after diagnosis. Approximately 50% of those with Multiple Sclerosis pursue most of the activities they engaged in prior to their diagnosis. In some cases, however, paralysis of different severities may make it necessary to use a cane, crutches, and other aids while walking. In a very small number of cases, the disease accelerates and may result in life-threatening complications.

CAUSES

The exact cause of Multiple Sclerosis is not known. An auto-immune association, possibly in a viral or environmental setting, has been suggested. The human T-lymphotropic virus (HTLV-1) has been proposed as another possible cause. The HTLV-1 virus is a retrovirus (a retrovirus is one which can transfer its genetic material into the DNA of the host cell – they are implicated in the aetiology of a number of cancers) that has been associated with other central nervous system disorders and certain blood malignancies. It is also suggested that an hereditary predisposition may be a factor, but it does seem that other factors need to be present as well.

It has been proposed that a Multiple Sclerosis "susceptibility gene" (MSSG) exists. There is, as yet, no definite genetic pattern that can be discerned.

HOMŒOPATHIC TREATMENT

Specifics to consider include *Avena sativa* in tincture, *Lathyrus* 3x, *Physostigma* 3x and *Hypericum* 3x. Constitutional prescribing is a must (as usual) and Murphy lists plenty of suggestions on page 425 (Diseases). As a time saving treat, here is a table showing my top four MS remedies and their differentials:

Multiple Sclerosis Remedies		
Remedy	**Comments**	**Modalities**
Causticum	Paralysis of single parts. Progressive loss of muscular strength, tearing pains. Weakness progressing to paralysis.	Raw and sore. >damp, wet weather. > warmth.
Gelsemium	Remedy action centred on the nervous system. Motor paralysis. Dizzy, drowsy, dumb, dull, droopy and trembling. Muscular weakness. Lack of co-ordination.	< damp weather < bad news. > stimulants.
Natrum mur	Great debility. Most weakness is felt in bed, in the morning. Weak and weary. Dry mucous membranes. Emaciation of the neck.	< lying down. < 10am. > cold air. > tight clothing.
Phosphorous	Inflammation of the spinal cord and nerves, causing paralysis. Suddenness of symptoms. Ataxia.	< touch. < warm food. > cool.

PARKINSON'S DISEASE

This is a slowly progressive disabling ailment, marked by tremor and increasing stiffness of the muscles. The disease, which occurs in all parts of the world, affects more men than women and is most likely to develop after the age of 35. The disease results from degeneration of the basal ganglia, an area of nerve cells at the base of the brain. The chief carrier of nerve signals in this area is the chemical dopamine, which is grossly deficient in Parkinsonian patients.

The cause of this deficiency is not known, but the discovery in 1983 that the chemical MPTP (a by-product of a synthetic form of heroin) could cause similar damage suggests that Parkinson's disease may have an environmental origin. Symptoms of the disease include excessive salivation, poor co-ordination, faulty body balance, tremors, and muscle rigidity. Shortening of muscles along the front of the neck tends to bend the head and spine forward.

It is one of the more commonly seen neurological conditions, occurring in about 1 in 400 of the population over 65. The signs and symptoms to look for in treating Parkinson's are those associated with tremor and those associated with rigidity. The tremor is quite typical and takes the form of a slow, coarse, regular, shaking of the fingers and limbs (and occasionally the head in my experience). It can produce a 'pill – rolling' movement of the thumb and forefinger. The tremor disappears during voluntary movement and reappears when the patient rests; so it is known as a Resting Tremor.

The rigidity however, is the most disabling feature of the disease. The patient is stiff and has poverty of movement, and this often means that initiating activity is the difficulty for them. Once initiated, an activity can be carried out, albeit rather stiffly and awkwardly, and the rigidity is associated with painfulness. Problem areas are walking, fastening buttons, shoelaces, writing (which has a very typical pattern of starting off fine and gradually getting smaller and less legible – a dead giveaway) and even speaking can be difficult as the smoothness of speech is lost.

The signs and symptoms to look out for are awkward movement; usually a kind of shuffling gait – the gait has a rhythm to it, changes in the voice (often an increase in pitch), stooped posture and a loss of facial expression. The latter can be very distressing for the sufferer and also their family. Other features include difficulty swallowing and a loss of intellectual functioning.

In the older literature we see Parkinson's disease described as 'paralyis agitans' – this means an agitating tremor and shaking – the key features of the disease, as we've seen. There are a number of aetiological possibilities for this disorder including trauma, drugs, carbon monoxide poisoning, viruses, and reaction to major tranquillisers (the latter known as Parkinsonian side effects). Conventional thinking suggests that there are increased risks from stress, arteriosclerosis, tumours, and in men over fifty.

CONVENTIONAL TREATMENT

The common understanding of treatment of Parkinson's is that the missing dopamine is replaced by giving L-dopa to boost the dopamine levels. As in all stuff to do with the brain this is an oversimplification – dopamine works in conjunction with acetylcholine in the area of the brain responsible for coordination of movement. These two chemicals have finely balanced opposing actions – so the reduction of dopamine is mirrored by an increase in acetylcholine. Consequently the 'balance' can be restored by using dopamine boosting drugs or by using drugs which block the action of the acetylcholine.

In general either of these approaches seem to have a beneficial effect on the problems associated with the rigidity, but are less effective at reducing the tremor. In practise the drugs are often given in combination. The common anticholinergic drugs include procyclidine, benzhexol and orphenadrine. Dopamine boosting drugs include levodopa, pergolide and apomorphine.

Levodopa, unfortunately is a drug with quite a few possible side effects; these include anorexia, nausea and vomiting, insomnia, agitation, hypotension, dizziness, tachycardia, arrhythmia, red urine, abnormal involuntary movements, hypomania, psychosis, depression, drowsiness, headache, flushing, sweating, gastro-intestinal bleeding, peripheral neuropathy and liver enzyme changes.

HOMŒOPATHIC TREATMENT

Remedies under consideration should include *Avena sativa*, as well as *Lathyrus Sativa* 3x to 30c, as well as more common remedies such as *Rhus Tox*, *Mercury*, *Zinc*, *Thuja* and *Conium*. For even more examples see Parkinson's Disease in Murphy (page 430). Some useful remedies are listed here:

ARGENTUM NITRICUM

Agitation and incoordination are keynotes of this remedy and therefore it's bound to be worth considering for this disease. Argentum nitricum has a 'hasty gait' – they actually seem to walk a little too fast. When you observe them you can see that they are using their momentum to carry them forward. They suffer from extreme uncontrolled tremor and are noticeably worse from any excitement...anger particularly, but any emotional upset may be an aggravating factor. It's said that Argentum nitricum is particularly susceptible to the phases of the moon, so it might be worth checking out whether the patient is notably angry, irritable, or restless at the new moon or full moon. They can overreact to practically anything – something you say, the weather, the temperature (generally they are worse for heat), or even to certain foods. This remedy is very sensitive to sweets; they crave them, yet they make them feel worse. *Argentum nitricum* also suffers from vertigo, which is not an uncommon concomitant to Parkinson's.

PLUMBUM METALLICUM

Look out for a history of working with lead or even with paint, which traditionally had a high lead content. This remedy has a staggering gait and is very, very clumsy. In *Plumbum metallicum* the tremors can be painful.

GELSEMIUM

Notable for tremor with weakness and fatigue, there can also be an aetiology which points towards the disease starting following an attack of influenza or viral infection – these are seen conventionally as possible causative factors in Parkinson's. The usual picture of *Gelsemium* applies – dizzy, drowsy, fatigue from the least exertion and heaviness in the limbs.

ZINCUM METALLICUM

In *Zincum metallicum* we see a sensitive nervous system; sensitive to light, noise, touch, smell and even to taste. This remedy has severe jerking of the lower limbs (twitchy and fidgety feet) and a shaking of the head. The legs are so twitchy they are even restless during sleep.

MERCURIUS

One of the possibilities for the aetiology of Parkinson's is mercury poisoning, the obvious suspect would be in dental fillings, but it has also been used in paint. They suffer from memory weakness, shaking, and tremors, and the usual *Mercurius* modalities apply – they're worse for a change in temperature (which can produce goose bumps) and for the least draught. Because of the likelihood of mercury fillings being a contributory factor there may be any of a multitude of mouth symptoms including fetid breath, ulcers, excess saliva and a yellow flabby tongue.

ALZHEIMER'S DISEASE

This is a progressive degenerative disease of the brain now considered a leading cause of dementia. It was first described by the German neuropathologist Alois Alzheimer in 1906. The incidence of the disease increases with advancing age, but there is no evidence that it is caused by the ageing process. There are over 75,000 cases in the UK at present and one in five people over 80 are affected, so you are highly likely to see it in clinic to some degree. It is the fourth most common cause of death in this country (after our old favourites heart disease, cancer and strokes).

The average life expectancy of persons with the disease is between five and ten years, although many patients now survive 15 years or more due to improvements in care and medical treatment. The cause of this disease has not been discovered, although palliative therapy is available. The ability of doctors to diagnose Alzheimer's disease has improved over the last ten years, but this remains a process of elimination and final diagnosis can be confirmed only at autopsy.

In my experience a specific remedy for Alzheimer's is *Ginkgo Biloba* – although it may only stabilise or slow down the pathology. Also worth considering would be *Alumina, Hyoscyamus, Arsenicum* and *Phosphorus.*

Hyoscyamus and Alzheimer's
One of the most disturbing features of Alzheimer's disease (and all dementia) is that there is often a degree of insight into the loss of function, especially in the early stages of the disease. Bear this in mind when treating dementia. There will be sadness and frustration. Hyoscyamus 'disturbs the nervous system profoundly-it is as if some diabolical force took possession of the brain' (Boericke). It causes mania of a quarrelsome and obscene manner. They are suspicious (with fear of poisoning), inclined to laugh at everything and also to run away. There can also be a deep stupor. Describe the picture of the remedy to anyone working with elderly, mentally infirm people and they will instantly recognise it as typical of Alzheimer's disease.

HEADACHES (SEE PAGE 28)

While some may be rooted in Nervous System pathology, headaches are all covered under the Musculoskeletal System.

FURTHER READING

John Ball **Understanding Disease**
Blackdown Publications
ISBN 0-85207-229-5

James Compton Burnett **The Best of Burnett**
B Jain Publishers
Book code B 3656

Lynne McTaggart **What Doctors Don't Tell You**
Thorsons
ISBN 0-7225-3124-2

C P Hart **Therapeutics of Nervous Disease**
B Jain Publishers
ISBN 81-7021-011-9

A L Blackwood **Diseases of the Kidneys and Nervous System**
B Jain Publishers
ISBN 81-7021-140-9

NOTES

NOTES

CONTENTS

THE DIGESTIVE SYSTEM

THE DIGESTIVE SYSTEM AND DIET

The digestive system is essentially a tube that is open at both ends. Consequently the lumen of the digestive system (the 'space' inside us) is an extension of the outside environment. Inside this system we meet the outside world more thoroughly than we realise.

The whole gastro-intestinal tract is a mucous membrane – and we need to be aware, as homœopaths, that this membrane will sometimes 'take on' pathology that the skin is unable to deal with. And vice-versa of course. This tract is complementary to the skin; they're both in some sense 'external' structures. So if there's a history of skin problems that have been conventionally treated (and possibly suppressed) that pathology can move inwards and manifest within the mucous membrane. This is a process that we also see occurring with the skin and the lungs – the internal manifestation of an 'external' disease that has been suppressed.

Don't be surprised therefore if you treat gastro-intestinal pathology and a skin eruption follows – this is a fairly common occurrence.

As a race we are supposed to have an intelligent but unconscious barrier at the 'point of origin' of this system – in other words in our mouth. Our senses of smell and taste are designed to prevent us from putting anything into the system that isn't good for us. We can see that this barrier is still in place for most animals (most of the time) – the likelihood is that most animals will not eat anything (natural) that is bad for them. However our culture has added a number of things to food to 'fool' that innate intelligence into eating artificial, or processed food, including:

- Salt.
- Spices.
- Flavourings.
- Colourings.
- Additives.
- Sauces.

These 'extras' fool us by making food pleasant smelling and tasty looking. Consequently many of our patients will have complaints that are diet-related…as does the population at large. Something like 50% of people in the western world die of heart-related illness; this is due to high cholesterol, high fat, and high salt diets. Factors that should not be part of our natural diet.

FUNCTION OF THE DIGESTIVE SYSTEM

The function of the digestive system is to transform unusable materials into something usable as fuel for the body. This is done by chemical and mechanical means. The easiest way to look at the system is to take one organ at a time.

MOUTH

The Salivary Glands secrete saliva, which aids mechanical digestion. Saliva contains:

- Mucus; which lubricates the bolus (the soft mass of chewed food.)
- Water; (99% of saliva is water) which dissolves the food for taste.
- Amylase; an enzyme that aids chemical breakdown of starch.
- Lysozyme another enzyme which is an antibacterial catalyst.

THROAT AND OESOPHAGUS

This system transports the food to the stomach (and prevents it from going down the trachea to the lungs). The throat and oesophagus use peristaltic action and the oesophagus has sphincters at either end ... the upper sphincter is the Oesophagus Sphincter and the lower one is the Cardiac Sphincter, which opens to the stomach.

STOMACH

The Cardiac Sphincter allows food into the stomach where it is processed both chemically and mechanically. The chemical process is controlled by gastric secretion from a number of cells in the folds of the stomach. The 'Big Four' types of cell are:

- **Parietal Cells:** which secrete Hydrochloric Acid that activates pepsin and disinfects the stomach.
- **Mucous Cells:** which releases mucous to protect the stomach wall.
- **Chief Cells:** which secrete Pepsinogen, which in an acid environment divides into pepsin. Pepsin is a remarkable enzyme; it helps to start the digestion of proteins by splitting them into peptones and can also act on pepsinogen to produce more pepsin.
- **Endocrine Cells:** which secrete gastrin into the blood to stimulate the activity of gastric juices.

The mechanical treatment of food in the stomach (Gastric Motility) is essentially a process that turns the bolus into chyme (chyme is the semi-liquid acid mass that is the form in which food passes from the stomach to the small intestine).

A series of peristaltic contractions occur in the stomach, at a rate of about three per minute (so any pains which occur at that sort of rate may well be traced to the stomach).

Gastric peristalsis also delivers the chyme to the small intestine (via the duodenum of the small intestine) – this is known as gastric emptying.

Various factors influence the rate at which this is done:

- Liquidity – highly liquid chyme increases the rate.
- Chyme in the duodenum automatically decreases the rate.
- High acidity in the duodenum decreases the rate.

- Fats in the duodenum decrease the rate.

The second, third and fourth factors in the list decrease the rate of gastric emptying to allow more time for digestion of chyme in the intestines. So we can easily see the factors that can lead to a feeling of *indigestion* … previously consumed food, acidic food and fatty food.

SMALL INTESTINE

The small intestine is where most digestion takes place. The inner lining, or mucosa, is folded and covered with tiny fingerlike projections called villi, a design that maximises the absorptive surface area of the intestine. Rhythmic contraction of the muscular walls moves food along while bile, enzymes, and other secretions break it down. Nutrients absorbed into the intestine's many blood vessels are carried to the liver to be distributed to the rest of the body.

Intestinal juice is secreted by the small intestine. It contains a number of enzymes; its function is to complete the process begun by the pancreatic juice. The mechanical pressure of food partly digested in the intestine stimulates the flow of intestinal juice.

Transport of the products of digestion through the wall of the small intestine may be either passive or active. Sodium, glucose, and many amino acids are actively transported. The products of digestion are thus assimilated into the body through the intestinal wall, which is able to absorb nutritive substances selectively, rejecting other similar substances.

The stomach and the colon or large intestine also has the ability to absorb water, certain salts, alcohol, and some drugs and crystalloids. Certain whole proteins are also believed to pass through the intestinal barrier. Intestinal absorption has another unique feature. Many nutrients are more efficiently absorbed when the body need is greater. The absorptive, extensively convoluted surface of the intestine amounts to 140 sq. m (1500 sq. ft) in an adult. The absorption is also aided by the length of the small intestine, 6.7 to 7.6 m (22 to 25 ft).

The water-soluble substances, including minerals, amino acids, and carbohydrates, are transferred into the venous drainage of the intestine and through the portal blood channels directly to the liver. Many of the fats, however, are re-synthesised in the wall of the intestine and are picked up by the lymphatic system which carries them into the systemic blood flow as it returns through the vena caval system, bypassing an original passage through the liver.

LARGE INTESTINE

Anchored in the abdomen by membranes called mesenteries, the large intestine is the final section of the digestive tract. Undigested material passes from the small intestine as liquid and fibre. In the large intestine, muscular segments called haustrae shuttle this material back and forth, mixing it thoroughly.

Cells in the smooth walls absorb vitamins, minerals, and water. Condensed waste, called faeces, leaves the body through the rectum.

EXCRETION

Undigested material is formed into a solid mass in the colon by reabsorption of water into the body. If colonic muscles propel the excretory mass through the colon too quickly, it remains semi-liquid. The result is diarrhoea. Insufficient activity of the colonic musculature, of course, produces a tendency to constipation. The stool is held in the rectum until excreted through the anus.

NEURAL REGULATION OF THE DIGESTIVE SYSTEM

The organs of the digestive system are regulated by the sympathetic and the parasympathetic nervous systems.

- The parasympathetic nervous system in general increases the gastric secretion and motility.
- The sympathetic nervous system in general inhibits the gastric secretion and motility.

There are three phases which are affected by these nervous systems:

1) Cephalic Phase: During this phase sight, odour and taste stimulate the medullary digestive centre (via the cerebral cortex and the hypothalamus).
2) Gastric Phase: Arrival of food in the stomach stimulates stretch receptor and chemoreceptor cells and thence the vagus nerve, (stretch receptor cells are found between muscle fibres and respond to stretching of those muscles by transmitting impulses to the central nervous system). Signals are passed via the Medullary Digestive Centre to the cardiac sphincter and smooth muscles in the stomach, increasing motility.
   The secretion of gastric juice is also stimulated. (In the cephalic phase 20% of the gastric juice is stimulated and in this phase the remaining 80%).
3) Intestinal Phase: The arrival of food in the duodenum of the small intestine is relayed via the receptor cells to the vagus nerve and initially Gastrin is secreted; later Gastric Inhibitory Peptide will decrease the secretion of Gastrin.

Definitions for this page
• The medullary digestive centre activates the Vagus nerve. • The Vagus nerve stimulates the secretion of gastric juice and pancreatic juice.

It is worth noting that the Intrinsic Nervous System also has a role in the process because the submucosal and myenteric plexi are 'directly' connected to the sympathetic and parasympathetic systems and increase Gastrin and motility respectively. This is known as the myenteric reflex – a reflex action of the intestine whereby a physical stimulus causes the intestine to contract above the point of stimulus and relax below it.

THE MOUTH

The issue of dental problems is one which is separate from the study of the digestive system, but it's probably worth looking at a couple of the more common disorders which manifest in the mouth. So here goes …

CANDIDA

This is a genus of yeast-like fungi that inhabits the vagina and the alimentary tract and can – under certain conditions – cause an infection. The infection is properly known as candidiasis, and commonly known as thrush. It appears in people who are debilitated and in babies who get it from the mother. The major sign is a cheesy white deposit that may be sore and/or irritable. There is a school of thought which sees recurrent or chronic candida as a precursor to more debilitating illness – possibly ME, so it as well to treat it seriously. There is no substitute for a well-observed diet with avoidance of sugar and alcohol, but helpful remedies include the *Candida nosode, Nitric acid, Kali mur* and *Borax.*

LEUCOPLAKIA

Is a pre-malignant condition found in the cheek or tongue where the mucous membrane looks raised, white and crinkly. Excessive smoking or drinking or ill-fitting dentures can cause it. Remedies to consider include *Thuja, Kali chlor, Lac-c, Sulphuric acid.*

ANGULAR STOMATIS

Also known as **Chelitis,** is an inflammation of the lips manifested by cracks in the corner of the mouth. This needs to be noted as it may indicate a vitamin B deficiency or it may indicate cancer of the stomach. It is a condition that is common in Parkinson's Disease. Top remedies are *Graphites, Nitric acid* and *Silica.*

DIVERTICULITIS

In some parts of the (descending) colon small pockets 'extend' through the wall; in essence a herniation of the mucous membrane. Each of these pockets is called a diverticulosis and of itself is not usually a problem. However if small bits of faeces go into the pockets and get stuck there, they can then harden and stomatise to become faecoliths. If the faecolith causes inflammation of the mucosal area this creates a case of diverticulitis. It is a real 'age thing'. In radiological surveys on healthy subjects diverticuli were found in 8% of the adult population under 60 and in 40% of those over 70.

SIGNS AND SYMPTOMS OF DIVERTICULITIS

Diverticulosis is likely to be a symptom-free condition; when inflammation commences (diverticulitis) there will be:

- Colicky pain on the left side.
- Pain on pressing the surrounding area.
- Ineffectual urging.
- Diarrhoea or constipation.
- Heavy rectal bleeding.

There may be a pattern of respite and relapse, and with chronic conditions it is possible that there will be some narrowing of the descending colon due to scar tissue (or abscesses or fistulas). Fistulas are an abnormal communication between two hollow organs or between a hollow organ and the outside world.

In diagnosis there can be some confusion between diverticulitis and IBS; but on investigation IBS has no visible pathology (ie. no diverticulosis).

CONVENTIONAL TREATMENT

It is worth noting that the diverticulosis is thought to be largely caused by increased pressure "from the inside out" in the colon. This can be attributed to a lack of fibre in the diet; our refined diets now have too little fibre and this lack of bulk means that the stool entering the colon is reduced. Consequently the 'transit time' is increased, the stool is more difficult to pass and therefore requires greater pressure of peristalsis. Over time this strain on the walls of the colon shows itself in these herniations. Consequently medical treatment may consist of advising a high residue or high fibre diet.

Various drugs may be prescribed including belladonna derivatives (Atropine, Propantheline, etc.) that help to inhibit the contractions, which can occur with diverticulitis and thus prevent the painful crampings. As diverticulitis has been associated with anxiety in the patient, Valium or Librium may be prescribed. Morphine-based painkillers are not usually used (because they increase the colonic pressure), but other painkillers may be prescribed.

There are a small minority of patients who will need surgery; this is an option when there is persistent bleeding.

As a first option however, the medical profession takes a natural approach. The most important factor seems to be the diet, which must be bulky in order to make the work of the colon easier. There have been studies in both America and this country which show that additionally, it is efficacious to introduce unprocessed bran into the diet. A typical suggestion would be to work up to four tablespoons a day of the bran (additional to diet) and allow the patient to increase the daily amount in response to cramps and pain. This regime has been found to be beneficial to those who have had surgery, increasing the effectiveness of the surgery, but more importantly it can even negate the need for surgery at all and leave the patient symptom free. In the acute phase of the disease it is likely that a relatively roughage free diet would ease the pain and discomfort.

HOMŒOPATHIC TREATMENT

The major remedies are shown in the table below. It is my experience that homœopathy can be very effective, but only in conjunction with dietary changes (and sometimes lifestyle changes too.)

Remedy	Comments	Modalities
Colocynth	Cutting, griping or intermittent pains, extremely severe with flatulence or diarrhoea. Followed by tenesmus. (sensation associated with desire to defecate.).	< anger, indignation > doubling up, pressure, warmth, head forwards.
Chamomilla	Pinching and twisting pain, soreness of the bowels, nausea.	< heat, anger, open air, night. >being carried, warm wet weather.
Nux vomica	Spasms and flatulence, pain as if the bowels and bladder were pressed upon with a cutting instrument. Irregularity in the action of the bowels, tendency to recur.	< morning after eating, touch, spices, stimulants, dry weather, cold > a nap, evening, at rest. damp, wet weather, strong pressure.
Iris versicolor	Severe flatulence. Try if other remedies fail.	< evening, night and rest >continued motion.
Belladonna	Paroxysms. Griping and sensation as if a ball were forming. Distension. Red face.	< touch, jar, noise, draft. >Semi-erect.
Veratrum album	Severe cramp, coldness of the whole body, flatulence, especially at night. Swelling and loud rumbling.	< night, wet, cold weather. > walking, warmth.

There are also a number of other remedies to consider, any number of acute remedies and constitutionally (in addition to *Nux Vomica*) one could think of *Lycopodium*, *Arsenicum*, *Plumbum*, *Bryonia* and *Mercury*.

IRRITABLE BOWEL SYNDROME (IBS)

This condition, also known as Spastic colon or Mucous colitis, is a incredibly common condition wherein there is recurrent abdominal pain and also constipation or diarrhoea. It can continue for many years without any apparent deterioration in health. There is no visible pathology in IBS (as distinct from Diverticulitis) and the symptoms are caused by abnormal muscle contractions in the colon. The cause is unknown but the syndrome has been associated with stress and anxiety, and may follow on from a severe infection of the intestine.

HOMŒOPATHIC TREATMENT

In psychological terms we would consider this type of patient to be an "anal worrier" and the condition can often be traced back to one event … so the aetiology may be a particularly interesting area to explore when taking the case. The patient may have an obsessive personality and fussy eating habits. Typically there may be an aversion to or aggravation from fruit, fried food and salads – in terms of remedies those outlined above for Diverticulitis form a good starting point when supported by well-selected constitutional treatment.

As this syndrome is so often confused with Diverticulitis it may be worth comparing and contrasting the two diseases:

Symptom area	Diverticulitis	IBS
Bleeding	Both diseases have bleeding.	
Age	Tend to be elderly.	Tend to be younger.
Bowels	> opening the bowels.	Bowel symptoms tend to change when in disease state.
Pain	Severe Colicky pain.	Pain in L or R iliac fossa (concave depression on the inside of the pelvis).
Diarrhoea	or constipation.	or constipation.
Diarrhoea		After breakfast.
Diarrhoea		Painless.
Diarrhoea		With rumbling and gurgling wind.
Defecation		After every meal.
Mental state	Natural concern and anxiety.	Fear of cancer of the bowel. Clear psychosomatic disorder.
First choice remedies	Lycopodium, Nux vomica	Sulphur.

HIATUS HERNIA

It isn't unusual for a hiatal (or "hiatus", both terms are equally correct) hernia to be 'silent', without any symptoms or complaints from the patient.

Whenever an organ pushes through a wall of the body cavity that encloses it, it is called a hernia. In men, the most common use of the term refers to the pushing of intestinal contents through the abdominal wall into the scrotal sac.

In a hiatal hernia, the stomach is pushing through the diaphragm, a sheet of muscle that separates the abdominal cavity from the chest cavity.

In general use, a "hiatus" means a gap, cleft or opening. Hiatus hernia is usually caused by an increased pressure within the abdominal cavity that may have been provoked by chronic coughing, straining, sudden physical activity, pregnancy, obesity, or as a result of some trauma.

Hiatus hernias occur in people of all ages and both sexes. Most usually it is seen in middle age and small hernias can be discovered in most people over the age of 50. In many cases the cause is not clear, but that doesn't affect the type of therapy needed; as for most asymptomatic cases, there is no treatment necessary for as long as there are no complaints. However, once complaints do become problematical both homœopathy and diet are important. As this problem is most common in men over 50, usually of the sedentary, but hard working business types; it is no great surprise that the top two remedies are *Lycopodium* and *Nux vomica.* Other prime candidates can be found in Murphy's Repertory – Diseases, Hernia, general (p.415).

DIABETES MELLITUS

Let's just start by making sure that we know the difference between diabetes insipidus and diabetes mellitus. The former is a rare metabolic disorder in which the patient produces large quantities of very dilute urine (I mean large quantities – up to five gallons a day). The disorder is due to deficiency of the pituitary hormone vasopressin (which regulates the reabsorption of water in the kidneys. Treatment is usually by administration of the missing hormone (usually nasally). Diabetes mellitus is what we normally mean when we say someone is diabetic. This is a disorder of carbohydrate mechanism in which sugars in the body are not oxidised because there is a lack of the pancreatic hormone insulin. The two disorders are completely unrelated.

Definitions for this page
Diabetes mellitus is a sustained and abnormal elevation of blood glucose concentration due to deficiency of insulin; the disorder also affects the absorption of fats, carbohydrates, water, proteins and electrolytes.

There are two 'common' divisions within the group known as diabetics: juvenile onset diabetes and late onset diabetes. Apart from the age difference there is often a difference of degree; the earlier diabetes has its onset, the more likely it is that the patient will require sustained medication.

There are a number of possible factors that might precipitate diabetes; here are some common indications:

SHOCK, STRESS, FRIGHT.

Possible remedy here would be *Natrum mur*. If it's a shock which the patient keeps reliving look at *Opium*.

OBESITY

Here again we see a difference between early and late onset diabetics. The early onset sufferers tend to be in their teenage years and are quite often thin; but late onset diabetes coming, as it does, at about 50 to 60 years (or later) the patient tends to be overweight.

HEREDITY

If one parent was diabetic there is a 50% chance of contracting the disease; if both parents had it the chance is 100%. There are 200 million diagnosed diabetics in the world. It is more likely to affect women and is more common in cities, which may indicate that there is a viral component.

SECONDARY DIABETES

Secondary, for example to cancer of the Pancreas.

SIGNS AND SYMPTOMS

- Fatigue – especially with weight loss.
- Appetite – increased (using proteins and fats to gain energy.)
- Thirst – obviously this is going to be a symptom of diabetes insipidus too.
- Polyuria – (peeing large amounts.)
- Itchy skin.
- Itchy genitals.
- White patches on the skin.
- Boils.
- Carbuncles.
- Impotence.
- Decrease in libido.
- Sugar in the urine.

COMPLICATIONS OF DIABETES

It is usual for diabetics to have a trace of glucose in the urine – this is to be expected. With poorly managed diabetes there can be large swings of glucose in the blood, and it is this that leads to the complications of diabetes.

GANGRENE

This occurs especially in the elderly in their extremities, often due to poor manicuring. The gangrene is a result of peripheral vascular disease that is caused by high levels of glucose and therefore ischaemia of the foot. (Ischaemia – inadequate blood flow). Gangrene can spread (in spite of treatment sometimes) and work up the leg, even to above the knee. Treatment is above the knee amputation.

Remedies for gangrene: *Calendula, Pyrogen, Gunpowder, Arsenicum, Lachesis, Secale, Carbo veg.*

DAMAGE TO THE NERVES

In diabetes there can be a general decrease in the sensitivity of the nerves or sometimes a tingling senstation. This damage to the nervous system can manifest in the eyes with retinopathy (ie. damage to the retina.)

INFECTIONS

Diabetics are more susceptible to skin infections than the general population; boils, carbuncles, fungus and candida to name but four.

FREQUENT COLDS

Again there is a greater susceptibility in diabetics.

DAMAGE TO THE KIDNEYS

Even to the extent of renal failure.

ARTERIOSCLEROSIS

Leading to Myocardial infarction, Ischaemic heart disease, or Angina.

BIRTHING DIFFICULTIES

It is a fact that diabetic women have larger babies than the general population, and this can lead to complications.

HYPO- AND HYPERGLYCAEMIA

There seems to be some confusion in many people's minds about these two conditions, so here is another table which compares and contrasts them:

	Hypoglycaemia	**Hyperglycaemia**
Blood Sugar	Lowered.	Raised.
History	No Food. Too much insulin. Unaccustomed exercise.	Too little or no insulin injection.
Skin	Moist.	Dry.
Blood Pressure	Normal or raised.	Lowered.
Respiration	Shallow or normal.	Kussmaul's respiration: rapid, deep, sighing respiration smells of pear drops.
Onset	Sudden and related to the last dose of insulin.	Insidious, over a period of days maybe.
Urine		Glycosuria (sugar in urine). Ketonuria (ketones in urine).
Treatment	Dextrose.	Insulin.
NB only diabetics who are being treated will become hypoglycaemic.		

CONVENTIONAL TREATMENT OF DIABETES

The medical profession views diabetes as an incurable disease, with clearly prescribed levels of treatment. For Type one diabetes, patients have to take insulin injections every day for life – this is to keep glucose levels normal. Most patients need from two to four injections per day.

Patients with Type two diabetes can maintain their glucose levels by diet alone, or by diet and oral medication.

HOMŒOPATHIC TREATMENT

Whilst it is worth bearing in mind that it would be foolish to claim to be able to offer a cure for diabetes, (not to mention potentially dangerous) there are any number of remedies that could help at a constitutional level – *Phosphorus, Lycopodium,* and *Carcinosin* among them. Many patients, especially in the earlier stages of diabetes might benefit from a remedy specifically to support and tone their pancreas – *Natrum sulph* and *Senna* are good examples. It would be extremely unwise to suggest that patients with diabetes change their conventional medication.

COELIAC DISEASE

This is a condition where the small intestine fails to absorb food. It affects 0.1 – 0.2% of the population and is due to a sensitivity of the intestinal lining to the protein gliadin, which is contained in gluten, from the germ of wheat and rye. This causes atrophy of the digestive and absorptive cells of the intestine. This disease manifests in children once they change to solid foods.

SIGNS AND SYMPTOMS OF COELIAC DISEASE

The severity of this disease can vary enormously. Some people may have the disease and be completely asymptomatic. It's worth noting that in babies the first signs and symptoms may appear after cereals are introduced to the diet. Possible key indicators include the following:

- Diarrhoea.
- Offensive stools.
- Failure to thrive.
- A 'malnourished' look.
- Stunted growth.
- Big belly and/or big face.
- … but small everything else.
- Insatiable hunger.

So, in this disease the villae in the small intestine can be denuded and atrophy; treatment is by a strict and lifelong gluten-free diet. You may hear this disease referred to as 'gluten enteropathy'.

Homœopathic remedies which are well worth considering are *Silica, Calc carb, Lycopodium,* and, as a 'specific' for coeliac disease, *Morgan Gaertner.*

CANCER OF THE COLON AND/OR RECTUM

This is one of the more common digestive cancers; conventional treatment is by surgery – re-section and colostomy. Cancers of the colon are slow growing but can spread to the liver or the lymph system. It has been noted that ulcerative colitis can 'lead' to cancer, as can polyps. One of the concerns about this form of cancer is that it can very easily metastasise. It tends to affect older people and starts with a change in bowel habit, anaemia and bleeding of the rectum.

SIGNS AND SYMPTOMS

- Weight loss.
- "Not feeling well".
- Intestinal obstruction (which may cause vomiting.)
- … therefore possibly fecal vomiting.
- Nausea.
- A 'blocked' feeling.

ACUTE SIGNS AND SYMPTOMS

- Visible peristalsis.
- Constipation with overflow (so the patient is constipated but there is a small amount of 'leakage'.)

Cancer of the rectum may be indicated by the symptom "sensation of incomplete opening". Remedies to consider include *Hydrastis, Arsenicum, Aluminum, Kali carb, Nitric acid, Sepia,* and *Ruta.*

WORMS

There are three major types of worms; Lumbricoides, roundworms; Teniae, tapeworms and Ascarides, threadworms. All three are in the Repertory – see Intestines, worms (p.1067). Roundworms are likely to be the result of contaminated food, so that may need investigating and a word with your local environmental health department might be in order. Threadworms become active in the late evening and at night and come out of the rectum at that time, followed, understandably by a sensation of a worm wriggling round the anus. Threadworms lay their eggs in the anus and are perpetuated by self-contamination. Symptoms include grinding of the teeth, irritability and much picking of the nose.

In children the big remedies are *Cina, Calc carb, Sulphur* and *Silica.* In general look at *Teucrium, Spigelia* and *Natrum phos.* Differentials between the three main remedies are as follows:

CINA

This is very possibly the number one remedy for worms; especially in children. Worms are often associated with behavioural problems such as hyperactivity, changes in appetite, changes to sleep pattern, even bedwetting. This remedy can help to alleviate all these changes as well as eliminate the physical problem. Here are a few symptoms to look out for:

- Intense 'voluptuous' itching of the anus.
- Gnawing pain in the stomach – sometimes associated with voracious appetite (but no weight gain.)
- Picking of the nose.
- Biting of the nails.
- Teeth grinding.
- Capricious behaviour.
- Bad breath.

SULPHUR

Another big remedy for worms, with severe anal itching (and burning) where the anus and surrounding area is red. The patient may well scratch the area until it bleeds. Possible clues to needing this remedy include:

- < Bathing.
- < Heat.
- History of previous skin infections – including nappy rash.

It may be worth considering that *Sulphur,* although an excellent remedy for worms, can sometimes aggravate the pain, itching, and heat in this condition. If the aggravation is very severe, *Arsenicum album* may help the situation.

TEUCRIUM

This is another frequently indicated remedy; notable for an itchy anus from worms and parasites. Symptoms are usually worse after bowel movements and also worse for the heat of the bed.

It has been my experience that worms are quite difficult to treat homœopathically, and as they are relatively easy to treat conventionally and can be very distressing, conventional treatment should be considered as an option.

ULCERS

The ulcers that you are most likely to come across in clinic are duodenal and gastric. Gastric ulcers are located on the lesser curve of the stomach or the lower oesophagus, whereas the duodenal ulcer is found in the duodenum. They are both caused by mechanical damage and diet (says conventional wisdom) but it is important to examine the personality as carefully as the pathology in cases of ulcers. Dietary factors to consider include drugs, alcohol, tobacco, aspirins, fatty foods, etc.

SIGNS AND SYMPTOMS

Both can present with pain; often a very specific pain that the patient can point to. Gastric ulcers tend to be worse shortly after meals, whereas duodenal ulcers cause pain a longer time after eating; maybe 2 – 4 hours afterwards. Both may be relieved by milk or mint. The patient with a duodenal ulcer may find blood in their stool; those suffering from gastric ulcers are more likely to have blood in vomit.

Gastric ulcers tend to become malignant and affect the older age group. Duodenal ulcers affect males predominantly (often between 40 – 55). The remedies to look at first will, of course, include *Nux vomica* and *Lycopodium*.

DIARRHOEA AND VOMITING

By far and away the most likely digestive system complaint you are likely to see will be diarrhoea and vomiting. Nonetheless, although very common, it is very important to have some idea of what's going on.

Diarrhoea and vomiting can be, among other things:

- a response to a toxin.
- a viral manifestation.
- alcohol abuse.
- drug induced.
- a response to deep x-ray therapy.
- parasites.

So ... before you start treating; ask yourself why is the patient like this? In the young and the elderly look out for dehydration. High fluid intake is usually to be encouraged in diarrhoea and vomiting. For all practitioners, vomiting with no nausea should be a red flag symptom. It is worth remembering that vomiting in the morning can be caused by pregnancy, alcohol abuse, too much spicy food, and anxiety. Vomiting at the end of the day may be due to an obstructive disease, and vomiting which makes the patient feel better may be due to ulceration.

CROHN'S DISEASE

This is a condition in which segments of the alimentary tract become inflamed, thickened, and ulcerated. It usually affects the Ileum (and can be called regional ileitis). Beware – it may mimic appendicitis! Chronically the disease can cause obstruction of the intestine – leading to pain, diarrhoea and malabsorption. Crohn's Disease is an autoimmune disease, occurs mostly in young adults, and conventional treatment is by surgery and/or steroids.

SIGNS AND SYMPTOMS

There may be long periods of time where this condition is 'inactive' – consequently there will be no symptoms of note. The disease pattern is of regular 'flare ups' however, with the following symptoms:

- Anaemia.
- Not being or feeling well.
- Poor appetite.
- Weight loss.
- Diarrhoea – up to 30, 40 times a day.

- Abscesses.

Remedies to consider are *Aloe, Arsenicum, China,* and *Merc-c.*

ULCERATIVE COLITIS

This is inflammation and ulceration of the colon and rectum. There is some dispute about the aetiology of this disease – it may well be another autoimmune disorder, and typically affects the 20 – 40 year age group.

SIGNS AND SYMPTOMS

- Grabbing pain.
- Urging to empty the bowel – up to 20 times a day.
- Mucosal, blood-streaked stool.
- Depression (hardly surprising)
- Significant weight loss.
- … and concurrent anaemia.
- Anxiety.

CONVENTIONAL TREATMENT

Conventional treatment is almost entirely drug based. It is always worth gaining some knowledge of conventional medication, especially so when working within this system as the majority of patients will be on some form of medication when they come to see you. Here are a few common categories of 'digestive drugs':

ANTACIDS

This is a group of drugs commonly prescribed for 'acid indigestion'. They work by neutralising the acid in the stomach, thus preventing inflammation.

One of the disadvantages of antacids is that they 'fool' the stomach into thinking that there is insufficient acid in the system. So, it produces more acid, and the patient needs more antacids – and so on.

Another disadvantage is that many antacids have, as their chemical basis, calcium carbonate. This is also the chemical basis of gallstones and kidney stones – so antacids may encourage the formation of stones.

Further disadvantages are that antacids can inhibit the absorption of other medication and they can disguise the symptoms of stomach cancer.

The common antacids are: Aluminium hydroxide, Calcium carbonate, Magnesium hydroxide and Sodium bicarbonate. Lovely.

ANTI-ULCER DRUGS

If antacid drugs fail sufficiently to do their job, or if the pathology is undiscovered for a long time, there may be a need for drugs to combat the ulcers formed by excess acids. There are two major types of anti-ulcer drugs; Proton pump inhibitors, and H2 blockers. Proton pump inhibitors block the enzyme system thus stopping the transport of hydrogen atoms and thence the secretion of acid. H2 blockers occupy the H2 receptors (histamine receptors) and thus prevent the production of acid. Overleaf is a table showing some of the main drug types and their side effects:

Type	**Example Drug names**	**Side Effects**
Proton Pump Inhibitors	Lansoprazole. Omeprazole.	Rashes, urticaria, pruritis, angiodema, alopecia, photosensitivity, diarrhoea, headache, nausea, constipation, flatulence, abdominal pain, dizziness, faintness, vertigo, somnolence, muscle and joint pain, blurred vision, peripheral oedema, increased sweating, impotence, loss of taste, candida, fever, bronchospasm, liver dysfunction, confusion, agitation, depression, hallucinations.
H2 Blockers	Cimetidine. Ranitidine.	Altered bowel habit, dizziness, rash, tiredness, reversible confusion, headache, blood disorders, muscle or joint pain, hypersensitivity, impotence
Other drugs	Antacids (see above). Bismuth. Cisapride.	

Until relatively recently drug treatment of ulcers was directed towards relieving symptoms, but since the discovery of a possible causative agent in *Helicobacter pylori*, cure is now aimed at in about a fortnight. *Helicobacter pylori (H. pylori)* is a spiral shaped bacterium that is found in the gastric mucus layer or adherent to the epithelial lining of the stomach. *H. pylori* causes more than 90% of duodenal ulcers and more than 80% of gastric ulcers. Before 1982, when this bacterium was discovered, spicy food, acid, stress, and lifestyle were considered the major causes of ulcers. The majority of patients were given long-term maintenance doses of acid-reducing medications, such as H2 blockers, without a chance for permanent cure. Since it is now believed that most ulcers are caused by *H. pylori*, appropriate antibiotic regimens can successfully eradicate the infection in most patients, with complete resolution of mucosal inflammation and a minimal chance of recurrence of ulcers.

THE LIVER

The liver is the largest internal organ of vertebrates, weighing 3-4 pounds. It is dark red in colour and is situated in the right upper quadrant of the abdominal cavity.

STRUCTURE

The liver appears as an outgrowth from the upper portion of the duodenum, just below the stomach. Unlike any other organ, the liver has two sources of blood supply: the hepatic artery carrying oxygenated blood from the heart and the portal vein carrying food substances from the stomach and intestines. These vessels enter the glandular tissue of the liver and break up into minute sinusoids (microscopic spaces between rows of liver cells.)

The general structure of the liver features two primary lobes. The left lobe is the smaller lobe, which extends out over the stomach and features the gastric impression. The right lobe is the larger of the two, being broader than the left and extending further down in to the abdominal cavity. The right lobe features the duodenal and renal impressions on its inferior (bottom) surface, accommodating the duodenum and right kidney. The liver is also shaped so that the front extends down into an edge, called the inferior margin, with the bottom surface slanting up sharply at the back. The gallbladder is on this bottom (back) surface.

FUNCTION

The liver and gallbladder are responsible for a number of functions. The main one relates to digestion, and the generation of digestive enzymes to be introduced into the small intestine.

The liver, however, also helps control metabolism and works with the body's immune system to combat rogue cells and organisms that threaten the body (in a process called "phagocytosis".)

Blood passes through the liver at a rate of about 1.4 litres (about 3 pt) per minute; at any instant, the liver contains about 10 percent of all the blood in the body. It also carries blood from the pancreas and spleen. The liver cells help the blood to assimilate food substances and to excrete waste materials and toxins, as well as products such as steroids, oestrogen, and other hormones.

The liver is a most versatile organ. It stores:

- Glycogen (the principal form in which carbohydrate is stored)
- Iron.
- Copper.
- Vitamin A.
- Many of the B-complex vitamins.
- Vitamin D.
- Anti-anaemic agents produced elsewhere in the body.

The liver produces Albumin and other proteins, including many of those essential to normal blood clotting (such as prothrombin and fibrinogen and the anticoagulant substance heparin.)

ACTION OF THE LIVER

In the liver, digested amino acids are deaminated; that is, their nitrogen is removed for use in the body. The liver can also use nitrogen to manufacture new protein (from carbohydrate or fat) and it can manufacture carbohydrate, from fat or from protein. Similarly, from carbohydrate or protein the liver can also make fat that it stores and later releases into the blood as free fatty acid, which can be burned for energy. So this is important to remember … when the body is short of fat, proteins or carbohydrates the liver will try to make up some of the shortfall.

Additionally the liver also synthesises cholesterol, and special phagocytes in the liver remove foreign bodies and bacteria from the blood. It secretes cholesterol, bilirubin (the breakdown product of haemoglobin) and many other substances, including enzymes. The liver also detoxifies many drugs.

In short, the liver:

- Helps digestion.
- Destroys red blood cells.
- Forms urea for the excretion of nitrogenous wastes.
- Forms fibrinogen used in blood coagulation.
- Stores glycogen & a range of vitamins.
- Helps in the metabolism of vitamins.
- Produces protective and antitoxic substances.
- The activities of the liver also generate a great deal of heat, affecting body temperature.

CIRRHOSIS

Cirrhosis is caused by chronic damage to the cells of the liver. Internal scarring (fibrosis) breaks up the normal structure of the liver. The undamaged cells multiply to form regeneration nodules. These nodules are inadequately supplied with blood, and as a result, over time, liver function is gradually impaired. In the United States about 30,000 deaths occur annually due to cirrhosis.

It is a long-term disease in which the liver becomes covered with fibre-like tissue, which causes the liver tissue to break down and become filled with fat. It is not unusual for cirrhosis to cause the liver to swell initially, the 'fatty liver', but then the liver shrinks as the fibrosis overtakes the attempts at regeneration … cirrhotic liver.

The word cirrhosis comes from the Greek meaning 'tawny' and this adequately describes the greyish-brown discoloration that occurs in the liver cells when they have been damaged. Cirrhosis is most often the result of long-term alcohol abuse, but can also be the result of malnutrition, hepatitis, or other infection. It can also occur as a result of heart failure.

Taken to its conclusion cirrhosis leads to liver failure (as may many other liver disorders), if there are not enough functioning cells to do the work of the liver.

SIGNS AND SYMPTOMS

As the most common (although not the sole) cause of Cirrhosis is alcohol – usually years of heavy drinking – so there may be a whole range of concomitant symptoms linked to alcoholism. Of course there are other symptoms as follows:

- Wasting due to the inability to form proteins.
- Spider naevi, dilation of capillaries in the skin of the face and neck.
- Gynaecomastia (male breast enlargement) which is caused by the inability to break down sex hormones, in particular oestrogen.
- Testicular atrophy and impotence for the same reason.
- Jaundice
- Coma… and subsequent death.

HOMŒOPATHIC TREATMENT

There are quite a few useful remedies for cirrhosis, as shown below:

Remedy	Keynotes	Modality
Sulphuric acid	Tremor, weakness. Hot flushes. Major Cirrhosis remedy.	< heat or cold in a.m. >lying on affected side.
Arsenicum iodatum	Irritating and corrosive discharges. Tubercular remedy.	
Aurum mur.	Indescribable weakness. Warts on tongue. Sycotic remedy.	Sensitive to heat. > wet weather.
Cardus marianus	Varicose veins. Haemorrhages. Oedema. Important liver remedy.	< stooping.
China	Abnormal excitement. Debility. Flatulence, bloating.	< slightest touch, eating > bending double, air.
Cuprum met	Spasms and cramps.	> perspiration.
Hepar sulph	Suppuration and sensitivity.	Liver < movement, touch.
Hydrastis	Thick, yellow secretions.	< bread, vegetables.
Iodum	Weight loss, goitre.	< quiet, right side.
Lycopodium	Liver remedy. Atony. Malnutrition. Craves warmth, pre-senility.	< right side, 4-8 p.m. >motion, warmth.
Mercurius	Tremors, glands up, bad breath.	< night, wet and damp.
Muriatic acid	Sepsis, high temp. and prostration.	< before midnight.
Phosphorus	Suddenness, degeneration.	< touch, twilight.

Remedy	Keynotes	Modality
Sulphur	Heat, relapse, offensiveness.	< rest, standing, warmth in bed > dry warm weather.

PORTAL HYPERTENSION

The liver has two blood supplies so if there is any blockage to the portal system (which is supplying the products of digestion straight from the digestive tract) pressure will start to back up. Blockages could occur because of tumour or cirrhosis. The backpressure will start to cause oedema and swelling of the gut. This can lead to significant swelling of the abdominal organs, especially the spleen.

This is not the only possible effect of blockage; there can also be a blockage to the blood, which can force it to take alternative routes. There are three possible alternatives:

- The oesophageal vein … the "top" of the system.
- The haemorrhoidal vein … the "bottom" of the system.
- The umbilical vein … in the middle of the system.

Re-routing blood to any of these three can cause venous distension and even rupture.

HOMŒOPATHIC TREATMENT

Some helpful remedies are shown here in this table.

Remedy	Keynotes	Modality
Aesculus	Sensation of fullness.	< walking > cool, open air.
Aloe soc.	Mucus and burning sensation in rectum.	< summer, heat, dry. > cool, open air.
Collinsonia canadensis	Sensation of sharp sticks in rectum. Haemorrhoids and constipation.	< mental emotion or excitement.
Leptandra virginica	Black, tarry stools, Yellow coated tongue.	
Lycopodium	Atony, malnutrition, right sided, Craves warmth, bloated.	> motion < 4-8 p.m
Nux vomica	Ratty. Soreness of abdominal walls. Itching haemorrhoids.	< after eating. > strong pressure.
Sulphur	Heat, relapse, offensiveness. Itching and burning of anus. Morning diarrhoea-drives out of bed.	< rest, standing, warmth in bed. > dry, warm weather.

HEPATITIS

Hepatitis is the term used to denote any inflammation of the liver; the word is derived from the Greek word Hepar, "liver."

The commonest cause of hepatitis is a viral infection of the liver. Chemical agents or poisons, drugs, bacteria or bacterial toxins, amoebic disease, and certain parasitic infestations may also cause hepatitis. Most cases of hepatitis recover, but a few progress to a chronic state that may lead to cirrhosis, a condition of progressive scarring.

In acute hepatitis, the disease is occasionally so severe that virtually all the liver cells are destroyed, and the patient dies of liver failure or by obstruction of the blood vessels leading from the liver.

There are three basic types of hepatitis; A, B and, cunningly, C. Hepatitis A virus infection is the most common form. It is spread primarily through fecal-oral contact, although improperly cooked contaminated shellfish, blood transfusion or possibly sexual activity may spread the infection.

Water and food-borne epidemics of Hepatitis A are common, especially in underdeveloped countries. Hepatitis A seems to be remarkably widespread in some countries where over three-quarters of the adult population appears to have been exposed. Hepatitis A virus can quickly spread through institutions and day care facilities where personal hygiene is less than adequate, particularly where there is not vigilance that people regularly wash their hands after using toilet facilities.

Hepatitis B Virus (HBV) is the second of the three viral agents that cause inflammation of the liver known as "hepatitis" or "diffuse hepatocellular inflammatory disease". In its most serious form Hepatitis B can become a chronic infection, or may cause liver cancer if left untreated. The hepatitis B virus can be passed from mother to unborn child, and is highly contagious through bodily fluids such as blood, semen and possibly saliva.

SIGNS AND SYMPTOMS

Hepatitis B Virus usually has a one to six week incubation period during which a certain antigen (immune response agent) circulates in the blood before symptoms of the illness develop. Hepatitis B may initially appear as influenza symptoms (fever, headache, eye-ear-nose-throat involvement, chills, tiredness, itchy rash, etc.), followed by nausea, vomiting and yellow discoloration of skin (jaundice). Because other diseases such as mononucleosis or chronic liver disease can cause similar symptoms, Hepatitis B may be difficult to diagnose.

Hepatitis B usually runs its course in four to eight weeks, except in some variations of the disease.

CAUSES

Hepatitis B is a form of acute viral hepatitis. It is usually transmitted by injection, transfusion of contaminated blood or blood products to hospital patients or by drug users sharing contaminated hypodermic needles. An increased risk to patients and personnel working in renal dialysis units has also been identified. Additionally sexual activity can spread the infection. However, hepatitis A virus is even more contagious than Hepatitis B. In many cases the source of infection with Hepatitis B virus is unknown.

The diagnosis of the three different types of Hepatitis (Hepatitis A, Hepatitis B, and Non-A, Non-B Hepatitis) is confirmed through antibody tests.

HEPATITIS C

Non-A, Non-B Hepatitis (Hepatitis C) virus infection is a little known infectious agent that can cause liver disease. Increasing evidence points to at least two separate viruses. In general, symptoms of this disease appear similar to Hepatitis B. It is usually spread through blood transfusions.

Remedy	Keynotes	Modality
Aconite	Intense thirst, bitter taste of food.	> open air. < warm room.
Arsenicum	Burning pain.	< wet weather. > heat.
Belladonna	Dread of drinking.	< touch, jar, noise, draught, afternoon.
Carduus marianus	Varicose veins. Haemorrhages. Oedema. Important liver remedy.	< stooping.
China	Abnormal excitement. Debility. Flatulence, bloating.	< slightest touch, eating. > bending double, air.
Lycopodium	Atony, malnutrition, right-sided, craves warmth, bloated.	> motion. < 4-8 p.m.
Natrum sulph	Brown, bitter coating on tongue.	< damp. > dry.
Nux vomica	Ratty, Soreness of abdominal walls. Itching haemorrhoids.	< after eating. > strong pressure.
Phosphorus	Suddenness, degeneration.	< touch, twilight.

THE GALLBLADDER

The gallbladder is a muscular organ that serves as a reservoir for bile, present in most vertebrates. In humans, it is a pear-shaped membranous sac on the undersurface of the right lobe of the liver, just below the lower ribs.

It is generally about 7.5 cm (about 3 in) long and 2.5 cm (1 in) in diameter at its thickest part; it has a capacity varying from 1 to 1.5 fluid ounces. The body (corpus) and neck (column) of the gallbladder extend backward, upward, and to the left. The wide end (Fundus) points downward and forward, sometimes extending slightly beyond the edge of the liver.

Structurally, the gallbladder consists of an outer peritoneal coat (tunica serosa); a middle coat of fibrous tissue and unstriped muscle (tunica muscularis); and an inner mucous membrane coat (tunica mucosa).

The function of the gallbladder is to store bile, secreted by the liver and transmitted from that organ via the cystic and hepatic ducts, until it is needed in the digestive process. The gallbladder, when functioning normally, empties through the biliary ducts into the duodenum to aid digestion by:

- Promoting peristalsis and absorption.
- Preventing putrefaction.
- Emulsifying fat.

GALLSTONES

The major disorder associated with the gallbladder is the presence of gallstones, varying in shape and size from a pea to a small pear. Built up from the constituent salts in the bile, they are most common in diabetic patients, in people of African descent, and in women; their presence increases with age. Two of the causative factors of gallstones are believed to be the presence of excessive amounts of substances such as calcium and cholesterol in the bile and the retention of bile in the gallbladder for a long period of time. The usual treatment for gallstones is surgical removal. Two naturally occurring bile salts, chenodeoxycholic acid and ursodeoxycholic acid, taken orally dissolve gallstones in some patients. Ultrasound treatment to shatter the stones also eliminates the need for surgery in some cases. The immediate remedies to choose from would include *Hydrastis* (as support in mother tincture) *Berberis* (also in mother tincture) and *Cholesterinum, Lycopodium, Natrum Sulph* and *Calc carb* in low potencies. Following this gentle intervention for a month or so, it would then be sensible to look at a deeper, more constitutional remedy.

CHOLECYSTITIS

Another common disorder of the gallbladder is cholecystitis, or inflammation of the organ, which is believed to be a result of the presence of highly concentrated bile and/or obstruction in the neck of the gallbladder, typically from a stone. Chronic cholecystitis is sometimes aggravated by streptococcal infection, to perforation and peritonitis. Causes of acute cholecystitis include typhoid fever, tumours, septicaemia and (naturally) gallstones.

SIGNS AND SYMPTOMS

Right-sided upper abdominal pain, raised temperature, nausea, aversion and/or aggravation from food, especially fatty food and pain < deep breathing.

The archetypal patient is fat, fair, forty, female and fertile.

Remedies to choose from:- *Pulsatilla, Calc carb.*

THE KIDNEYS

There are (usually) two kidneys, which lead physiologically to the Ureter, the Bladder and the Urethra.

STRUCTURE

In humans the kidneys are situated in the region of the loins, one on each side of the spine, and are embedded in fatty tissue. They are bean-shaped, possessing a convex outer border and a concave inner border. The inner border presents an indentation, the hilus, where the blood vessels enter and leave.

In front is the renal vein carrying blood from the kidney; behind it lies the renal artery carrying blood to the kidney.

THE FUNCTION OF THE KIDNEYS

- To control the water balance of the body.
- To control the pH of the body.
- To produce Erythropeitin, which increases the production of the red blood cells.
- To convert vitamin D into more active substances.

Important aside
It is worth remembering what vitamin D is for. This vitamin is necessary for normal bone formation and for retention of calcium and phosphorus in the body. It also protects the teeth and bones against the effects of low calcium intake by making more effective use of the calcium and phosphorus available.

Also called the sunshine vitamin, vitamin D is obtained from egg yolk, liver, tuna, and vitamin-D fortified milk. It is also manufactured in the body when sterols, which are commonly found in many foods, migrate to the skin and become irradiated.

Vitamin D deficiency, or rickets, occurs only rarely in tropical climates where sunlight is abundant, but it was once common among children of northern cities before the use of vitamin D-fortified milk. Rickets is characterised by deformities of the rib cage and skull and by bowlegs due to failure of the body to absorb calcium and phosphorus. Because vitamin D is fat-soluble and stored in the body, excessive consumption can cause vitamin poisoning, kidney damage, lethargy, and loss of appetite.

Other functions of the kidneys are:

- To produce urine.
- To excrete waste products.
- To produce Renin, which ensures that the blood pressure to the kidneys remains constant.

One of the most common collections of symptoms that we will see in practice that indicate kidney problems is an abnormal volume of urine. This may manifest in a number of ways, I have classified them under the medical terms appropriate, but it will be obvious how these symptoms may be described:

OLIGURIA

This is a reduction of urine output to less than 500 ml/day. The minimum obligatory output volume is around 400 ml/day. There can be a variety of reasons for Oliguria; it may be that the patient isn't drinking; or has had a severe shock; or it may simply be kidney dysfunction.

ANURIA

This is a reduction of the urine output to less than 250 ml/day. This could indicate chronic or acute renal failure or trauma to the kidneys. Obviously either of the above conditions would be alarming to the patient (hopefully) as they can lead to retention of toxins as well as dehydration.

Treatment to consider for either of the above conditions would include:

- Checking that the patient actually is drinking properly.
- Testing for dehydration (To test for dehydration pinch the skin. If it is dehydrated the 'pinch' stays and the skin doesn't return to normal).
- The usual treatments for shock.
- Immediately sending them to A & E or their GP.

HOMŒOPATHIC TREATMENT

Remedies to consider for either of the above conditions would include:

- *Arnica*, if there is trauma or shock as aetiology.
- *Aconite* if the modalities indicate. There may be shock, but also anxiety, fear of death and hot, dry skin.
- *Carbo Veg* if the patient is evidently in the last stage of disease; the skin would be cold (and sweaty) to the touch.
- *Urinum humanum* where urine is very scanty, thick deep brown and very offensive.

Chronic or acute renal failure could be very serious; certainly as the three main constituents of the blood build up in the body (water salt and urea) one would expect oedema, hypertension and uremia to occur. For the uninitiated uraemia is, quite simply, excess amounts of urea and other nitrogenous waste compounds in the blood. This would lead to nausea, vomiting, lethargy, drowsiness and eventually death. In complete renal failure (which anuria could indicate) coma can be expected within a week and death within two. The main remedy for uraemia is *Urtica Urens*, which "favours elimination" (Boericke) and is indicated if the patient has been stung by a bee prior to this problem (Murphy). Burnett discovered *Urtica urens* and cured a very severe case of uraemia with it. Also consider *Lycopodium* and *Hedeoma* (Pennyroyal.)

POLYURIA

This is the production of excessive urine, which could be indicative of either diabetes insipidus (or mellitus) as well as of kidney disease. Try to remember that increases in urine production can also indicate anxiety… . especially in young children; remembering this could save you a lot of time. This condition can also be found where there has been abuse of alcohol and/or cannabis.

NOCTURIA

Passing urine at night. This may indicate that the kidneys are having problems concentrating the urine. Top remedies would include:

- *Calc Fluor* — Everything is worse at rest and change of weather
  Better for heat.
- *Lycopodium* — Red sand in urine, < 4 – 8 p.m., back pain, urinating.
- *Spigelia* — Sensitive to touch, chilly, > lying right side.
- *Sulphur* — Involuntary passing of urine at night (enuresis).
  Burning in urethra during and after micturition.
  Mucus and pus in the urine.
  Great quantities of colourless urine.

In general terms it is worth checking urine for a number of factors if you are concerned about the function of the kidneys. (Or at least get your patients to check for you.) Check for concentration, colour, casts, deposits, proteins (these can be observed by 'strands' in the urine), sugar (yes there is an easy way to test for sugar… but it's probably better to check your own urine than somebody else's) and finally smell.

Blood in the urine clearly indicates damage (possibly of recent trauma) or dysfunction.

URINE COLOURS

As an observable variable in the case, and therefore as a sign of progress (or otherwise), knowing about the colour of your patient's urine might be very useful. Here are some examples of colour changes and what that might indicate. Long term changes in the colour of the urine should be a cause for concern and medical advice may well be very important.

- Red colour may be beetroot (ditto in the stool) there is even a name for this… beeturia.
- Red colour in new-borns is not uncommon and may just be urates.
- White/milky deposits = phosphates, possibly phosphoric acid.
- Yellow/green may be caused by Vitamin B tablets or bile.
- Red/brown may follow crush injuries. This can indicate blocked kidneys – possibly leading to complete renal failure.

RENAL FAILURE

The signs of renal failure are many and obvious, but just so you don't overlook them in practise here's a list to memorise:

- Flushing of the face.
- Increased BP.
- Congestive Cardiac Failure… and then lowered BP.
- Irregular pulse.
- Offensive breath, smelling of urine.
- Nausea, vomiting and diarrhoea.
- Hiccoughs.
- Skin becomes dry and scaly.
- Skin becomes itchy.
- Skin becomes yellow/brown.
- Cerebral oedema.
- Muscle twitching.
- Coma… leading to death.

NEPHRITIS

This is an inflammation of the kidney and is one of the commonest kidney diseases. Its chief characteristics are the appearance in the urine of such elements as albumin, (a condition known as albuminuria), red and white blood cells; and hyaline or granular casts, all revealed by microscopic examination of the urine.

Nephritis is a general term for inflammatory diseases of the kidney. Although many types of nephritis exist, the most common form is glomerulonephritis, or Bright's disease. In the western world, nephritis ranks high among the diseases that are a direct cause of death. Patients with acute nephritis generally recover, particularly children. A small percentage of cases result in chronic nephritis, which tends to be a progressive disease that gradually destroys the kidney.

Patients with acute nephritis often have a history of a streptococcal infection such as 'strep throat' a few weeks before the onset of nephritis. The disease is characterised by fatigue, appetite loss, facial puffiness, abdominal or flank pain, and scanty, smoky, dark urine.

Chronic nephritis usually presents no symptoms, but the urine will be found to contain albumin and, on microscopic examination, red blood cells. When there is an advanced destruction of kidney tissue with grossly impaired kidney function, patients may develop high blood pressure and die of kidney or heart failure.

In recent years, techniques such as dialysis have been successful in removing poisons that accumulate in the blood of patients with kidney failure. Improvement in kidney transplantation techniques has given hope to patients in the last stage of nephritis.

HOMŒOPATHIC TREATMENT

Here are a few suggestions for remedies. It should be borne in mind that this can be a painful and degenerative disorder, so swift and accurate homœopathy is needed, or a referral to a medical specialist.

- *Ocimum canum* with pain present on the right side.
- *Arnica* with the usual modalities.
- *Kali chlor* one of the great kidney remedies. Chronic conditions.
- *Terebinthina* oedema, drowsiness, strangury (severe pain in the urethra.)

KIDNEY TRANSPLANTS

A single kidney is sufficient to keep its recipient healthy because it will enlarge to function for the whole body. Kidney transplants are more straightforward than heart, liver or lung transplants, and 80 to 90 percent are successful. If the kidney is rejected, the patient can return to dialysis and, if otherwise healthy, undergo a second transplant surgery.

NEPHROSCLEROSIS

This is a hardening of the small arteries supplying the kidney and is a disorder characterised by the presence of albumin, casts, and occasionally white or red blood cells in the urine; it usually accompanies hypertensive vascular disease. Its fundamental lesion is a sclerosis of the small arteries of the kidney, with secondary atrophy of the glomeruli and pathological changes in the interstitial tissue. Aside from indicated remedies it might be appropriate to look at those that we normally consider for circulatory disorders:

Artery Organ Remedies: *Equisetum, Lobelia inflata, Cactus, Baryta carb, C-C-C Combination remedy*

RENAL CALCULI

Kidney stones may form in the kidney or renal pelvis from crystals deposited from the urine. They are composed mostly of calcium oxalate. Infection or obstruction may play a part in their formation. Sometimes they occur when the level of blood calcium is abnormally high, as may be the case when the parathyroid glands overproduce urine. Occasionally, stones may develop when the blood level of uric acid is too high, usually from over-consumption of meat. Excessive dietary intake of calcium and oxalate and low fluid intake have also been associated with formation of stones. In most cases, however, the cause is not known.

Stones may cause bleeding, secondary infection, or obstruction. Small kidney stones tend to travel down the ureter toward the bladder; their movement is usually accompanied by severe pain. Colic caused by stones usually requires one or more injections of narcotics for relief. The pain may develop suddenly after muscular exercise. Once a stone drops into the bladder, it may be passed with the urine unnoticed, and the pain ceases. If the stone is too large to pass, treatment is necessary, either with surgery or with lithotripsy, a procedure that uses shock waves generated outside the body to disintegrate the stones.

HOMŒOPATHIC TREATMENT

Kidney stones can be extremely painful. These remedies can be a great help, but appropriate pain relief (whether homœopathic or conventional) is often the greatest need.

- *Berberis vulgaris* The Kidney organ remedy par excellence, always consider.
- *Benzoic acid* Strong smelling urine, dark urine, joints crack.
- *Calc carb* Dark brown, sour, fetid urine… abundant with white sediment.
- *Pareira brava* Urinary system organ remedy. Pain going down thighs, constant urging, great straining, male remedy.

I would urge you to read Anshutz; "New, Old, and Forgotten Remedies" on *Calcarea renalis praeparata*. This is a remedy he made from one of his own Kidney Stones. He suffered terribly from stones and said of the remedy "It is true, the most suitable homœopathic remedies afforded me relief; the incarceration of calculi in the ureter especially was relieved by *Nux*; but they were unable to put a stop to the formation of calculi; this result was only attained by the preparation of *Calc. ren.*"

NATURAL HEALING FOR KIDNEY STONES

NUTRITION

Kidney stones (Calcium oxalate) occur, in the vast majority of cases, because of a double nutritional deficiency. Adequate daily supplements of the two deficiencies may be enough to rid the body of the stones. The two most commonly missing dietary elements are magnesium and vitamin B6.

Scientists Dr. E L Prien and S F Gershof (Harvard University) studied the use of these two supplements in a population of 36 patients who had all formed at least two kidney stones. Over the five year period of the trial 30 patients either had no further stone recurrence or markedly decreased recurrence (American Journal of Clinical Nutrition, 1967.)

Further studies show that 89% of the patients benefited from the treatment and 79% found "complete protection". Dr's Prien and Gershof stated "A number of patients having become free of stones stopped treatment and began having stones again within a few weeks, only to become free of stones again when they resumed treatment" (Journal of Urology, 1974.)

The Harvard team used 300 mg of magnesium (actually less than the RDA, which is 350 mg) and 10 mg of B6 (five times greater than RDA.)

Magnesium makes the urine more solvent with respect to oxalates; with greater solvency the fluid can hold crystals in solution with less risk of precipitation or aggregation; that is the clumping together of particles that causes 'stone formation'.

Vitamin B6 on the other hand has no effect on the solubility of oxalate in the urine but appears to control the body's production of oxalic acid and therefore limits the amount reaching the kidneys.

LUPUS ERYTHEMATOSUS

This is a chronic disease originally identified by the rash it caused but is now known to involve the internal organs in many cases. Lupus strikes women nine times as often as men. The disease is thought to be a result of the malfunctioning of the immune system. The blood of a lupus patient contains antibodies against many normal tissue components. Damage caused by these antibodies produces symptoms that can include the characteristic butterfly rash on the face, arthritic joint disease, heart damage, shortness of breath, and impaired kidney function. Lupus follows an irregular course of remissions and flare-ups, but is often incapacitating. Allopathic treatment is rest and drugs – nonsteroidal anti-inflammatories, antimalarials, or corticosteroids.

Remedies include *Lycopodium, Arsenicum, Nitric acid* and *Thuja.*

CYSTITIS

Cystitis is an inflammation of the bladder, usually from bacterial infection originating in the urethra, vagina, or in more complicated cases, the kidneys, this can sometimes be traced to stagnation of the urine, (e.g. in pregnancy).

Cystitis may also be caused by irritation from crystalline deposits in the urine or from any condition or urologic abnormality that interferes with normal bladder function. Symptoms include painful or difficult urination, urinary urgency, and, in some cases, cloudy or bloody urine. Allopathic treatment is primarily with antibiotics.

HOMŒOPATHIC TREATMENT

In acute cases homœopathy can be a fantastic and rapid relief. In recurrent or chronic cases it is really important to try and find out the underlying cause, and deal appropriately with that. The following are good acute remedies:

- *Cantharis* Pains < before micturition.
- *Apis* The last drops tend to burn.
- *Uva ursi* Slimy urine, burning.
- *Sarsparilla* Pain < end micturition.
- *Chimaphila umbellata* Cloudy urine, cancer of the uterus.
- *Medorrhinum* Fishy smell.

ENLARGED PROSTATE

This occurs in men at a percentage rate commensurate with their age (ie. it occurs in 60% of 60 year olds, 70% of 70 year olds, etc.). The prostate can enlarge as a result of benign or malignant problems. When it enlarges it presses on the urethra and thus obstructs the flow of urine.

Symptoms include hesitancy and urging and then only a few drops... "dribbling incontinence"

Eventually the prostate completely occludes the urethra and then complete retention of urine occurs. Consequently the urine can flow back to the kidneys – hydronephritis – and destroy kidney tissue. Ultimately this leads to kidney failure.

Remedies include:- *Calc carb, Thlaspi bursa pastoris, Fraxinus americana* and *Sabal serrulata.*

Problems with the prostate are associated with lack of zinc. This can be taken prophylactically in the form of supplements or pumpkin seeds.

FURTHER READING

Dr Douglas Borland **Homœopathy in Practice**
Beaconsfield
ISBN 0-906584-06-X

Dr Donald Foubister **Tutorials on Homœopathy**
Beaconsfield
ISBN 0-906584-25-6

David Hoffman **The New Holistic Herbal**
Element Books Ltd.
ISBN 1-85230-193-7

E A Farrington MD **Clinical Materia Medica**
B Jain Publishers
ISBN 81-8056-194-1

F Bernoville **Diseases of the Respiratory and Digestive System of Children**
B Jain Publishers
ISBN 81-7021-389-4

Jill Wright **Herbalism: Digestive disorders**
B Jain Publishers
ISBN :81-8056-150-X

NOTES

CONTENTS

THE CARDIOVASCULAR SYSTEM

The heart is the muscle that pumps the blood. To locate your heart (unless you are a politician) find the junction of the sternum and the ribs; the heart is two fingers breadth above that point. It lies slightly more to the left than to the right, is conical in shape and about the size of a closed fist.

Above the heart are blood vessels, below it the diaphragm, behind it the oesophagus, trachea and bronchus. It is protected at the front by the sternum and intercostal muscles. The lungs lie on either side of the heart.

There are three layers of the heart muscle as shown in this table:

Layer	Name	Function
Outside	Pericardium	Reduces any friction of the heart with surrounding organs and tissue, particularly the lungs.
Middle	Myocardium	This is the muscle of the heart. It is constructed like a trellis which enables great elasticity.
Inside	Endocardium	Smooth 'low friction' tissue called endothelium. This is flat and smooth and therefore less resistant to flow of fluid.

There are several conditions you may be familiar with that are specific to these areas, notably:

- Pericarditis which is inflammation of the pericardium (often accompanied by accumulation of fluid)
- Myocardial Infarction which denotes death of the myocardium
- Endocarditis which is where the smooth cells become 'rough'

The flow of blood through the heart can initially appear complicated and difficult to remember, but this process is basic physics allowing the heart to pump on average some 100,000 times a day and managing to move the blood around the body despite some of the cavities only containing a few teaspoons full of blood.

The following table sets out the flow of blood through the heart.

De-Oxygenated	FLOW	Oxygenated	FLOW
	From the body to superior vena cava to right atrium to right ventricle to pulmonary artery (the only artery in the body to contain deoxygenated blood) to the lungs		From the lungs to pulmonary veins to the left ventricle to the aorta to the body

Valves	TRICUSPID Prevents backflow from the right ventricle into the right atrium.	Valves	AORTIC Prevents backflow from the aorta into the left ventricle.
	PULMONARY Prevents back flow from the pulmonary artery to the right ventricle.		MITRAL Prevents back flow from the left ventricle into the left atrium.

The heart's own pacemaker and electrical system govern all the contraction and relaxation. In effect the 'top half' of the heart contracts followed by the contraction of the bottom half. It's important to know something about this process because the electrical processes of the heart are often used as a diagnostic tool – the electrocardiogram.

In brief a whole cycle takes, on average about 0.8 seconds. This "average" allows us to predict an average bpm (beats per minute) of about 75 (60 seconds divided by 0.8 for the non-mathematical). Obviously there can be a large variance in this time as the whole system responds to the demands placed upon the heart by the body – for example if you are doing some exercise the demand is going to be greater.

The increases in the heart rate are governed by the sympathetic nervous system. If there is a problem in this area it is clinically known as Tachycardia.

Decreases in the heart rate are governed by the Para-sympathetic nervous system and clinical problems are called Bradycardia (less than 50 beats per minute).

THE HEART

These diseases are laid out in no particular order. Of necessity some of the descriptions of the pathology are brief and simple, however they are a good starting point. The remedies cited are merely guidelines for your thought processes. There are no substitutes for careful constitutional or acute prescribing.

CARDIAC FIRST AID

If a patient falls to the floor in your treatment room, and you're sure they're not just worshipping your skills as a homœopath, these are the signs and symptoms to look for:

- Collapse
- Colour is likely to be at the blue/purple end of the spectrum
- Breathing, or more accurately lack of it…check the rise of the chest
- Pulse may be absent, check if there is a discernible pulse at the carotid or the wrist. If not, they have heart failure.

The first thing to do is **call an ambulance**. Even if you can do First Aid, you'll still need someone to help out; then lay him or her on a flat hard surface (if they haven't already obligingly fallen on one).

A Open airway by putting the head back, check the mouth is clear

B Check breathing

C Check circulation…carotid pulse

ADMINISTER FIRST AID

To recap: You should administer two breaths followed by fifteen heart massages, and continue to repeat, **checking after each cycle that they are still not breathing.**

Ideally you should do a first aid course, check for your local St. John's Ambulance Division or Red Cross Society both of whom offer comprehensive training.

CAUSES OF ACUTE CARDIAC FAILURE

There are a number of common causes for acute heart failure:

- Severe damage to an area of heart muscle due to a lack of blood, this is known as Ischaemia, and may be caused by a sudden closing of one of the larger coronary arteries.
- Pulmonary embolism, is where a blood clot is lodged in the pulmonary artery, this may be characterised by severe pain in the chest, coughing up blood and sudden death.
- Acute toxic Myocarditis; inflammation of the muscular walls of the heart.
- Severe cardiac arrhythmia.
- Rupture of one of the chambers of the heart.
- Severe malignant hypertension.

HOMŒOPATHIC TREATMENT

Remedy	Characteristics
Arsenicum	Mental distress, great anxiety, restlessness, thirst (small sips). Cold, burning pain in the chest, fear of death (with some justification it has to be said)
Antimonium tart	Cyanosis, exhaustion, hopeless and depressed, white tongue.
Carbo veg	Collapse, cold and clammy, dull and confused, want of air, pale.
Oxalic acid	INTENSE exhaustion and numbness, mottled cyanosis, wants to keep still, pricking pains in the chest.

CHRONIC CARDIAC FAILURE

This has (inevitably) a slower development and initially no symptoms, the causes include:

- Chronic hypertension
- Myocardial fibrosis
- Valve disease
- Lung disease
- Anaemia
- A history of previous acute failures
- Degeneration due to old age
-

HOMŒOPATHIC TREATMENT

Remedy	Characteristics	Differentiation
Lachesis	< lying left side, < into and after sleep. Tremor, dull, confused and suspicious, cyanosed.	Constriction.
Naja	< lying left side, < into and after sleep. Tremor, dull, confused and suspicious, cyanosed.	Stitching pain.
Lycopus	Tumultuous throbbing in the chest, < lying on the right side, < food and smell of food.	
Laurocerasus	Bluish appearance of the lips, dyspnoea, cold, < exertion.	

In practise you will be seeing patients who come with a diagnosis from our friends in the conventional sphere, this short section is designed to give you a quick guide to some of the more common diagnoses and their meaning.

RIGHT-SIDED CARDIAC FAILURE

This is also know as Congestive Cardiac failure.

Right-sided cardiac failure may be due to any or all of these factors:

- Resistance to blood flow through the lungs
- Weakness of the myocardium
- Valvular problems, which can be roughly divided into:
- Stenosis (narrowing), or
- Incompetence (flow-back)

HOMŒOPATHIC TREATMENT

Remedy	Characteristics
Crataegus	For myocardial weakness, increased pulse, oedema, cyanosis.
Lactrodectus	Valvular lesion, numbness of the left arm and hand.

LEFT-SIDED CARDIAC FAILURE

This is caused by one or more of the following:

- High systemic BP
- Incompetence of the mitral or aortic valve
- Stenosis of the mitral or aortic valve
- Myocardial weakness

HOMŒOPATHIC TREATMENT

Remedy	Characteristics
Spigelia	< touch, motion, noise, turning. > lying on right side with head high.
Digitalis	< sitting erect after meals. > empty stomach, open air.

ISCHAEMIC HEART DISEASE

Ischaemia is the term denoting inadequate flow of blood to a part of the body. In the case of the heart this may be due to narrowing of the coronary arteries (caused by plaques) and/or thrombosis (thrombosis is a condition where the blood turns from liquid into solid and clots, thereby closing part of the artery). If the arteries are narrowed this will lead to Angina pectoris. If they are occluded (closed) there will be myocardial infarction.

In Angina pectoris the narrowing of the artery means that there is insufficient capacity for blood supply to allow exercise, therefore exercise leads to pain in the chest.

HOMŒOPATHIC TREATMENT

Remedy	Characteristics
Aconite	Fear of death, restless but movement, <may be well indicated for the first ever attack but then of less use.
Cactus	Fear of eventual death, increasing tightness around the chest.
Arsenicum	Acute, distressing, burning pain.
Spigelia	Shooting pains followed by numbness.

MYOCARDIAL INFARCTION

In chronic Ischaemic disease the infarcts are small but may eventually collectively lead to weakness of the myocardium and thence to heart failure.

In acute Ischaemic disease the infarcts may be larger and thus disrupt the heart's activity. Death may occur.

RHEUMATIC HEART DISEASE

Following Rheumatic Fever, the heart becomes inflamed and oedematous. On healing there can be formation of fibrous areas that particularly affect the valves causing Stenosis and Incompetence. Also fibrous thickening of the pericardium may restrict the expansion of the heart.

CARDIAC ARRHYTHMIAS

Simply, this is where the heart is contracting in a disorderly manner; there are a couple of 'subsets' of Cardiac arrhythmias:

ATRIAL FIBRILLATION

This is where the pumping of the heart is ineffective and the stimulation of the AV node is disorderly. In this case an adequate circulation can still be maintained. Causes include Ischaemic Heart Disease, Degeneration due to old age, Thyrotoxicosis, and Rheumatic Heart Disease.

How to read an ECG
For the more technically minded, the electrical impulse in the heart originates in the sino-atrial node. This impulse spreads across the atria to the atrio-ventricular node. This causes the atria to contract and this process is indicated by the P wave on electrocardiographs. The electrical impulse is then conveyed down and into the ventricles by the bundle of His (the bundle of His is known in some texts as the atrio-ventricular bundle) and then ventricular contraction occurs. This is represented on an ECG by the Q-R-S complex. There is also a T wave which indicates that part of the cardiac muscle has relaxed before the cycle commences again.

Homœopathic Remedies to consider include *Digitalis, Argentum nit* and *Gelsemium*.

VENTRICULAR FIBRILLATION

This occurs when the pumping action of the ventricles is disrupted. If this cannot be reversed quickly it can be fatal. The condition is characterised by an increase in the heart rate (Tachycardia).

Homœopathic remedies include *Glonoine* and *Iberius amara*.

HEART BLOCK

If there is an increase in the delay between atrial and ventricular contractions, the heart rate may descend to 35 bpm (Bradycardia). In this state the heart cannot respond to sudden demands, causes include acute Ischaemic heart disease, Myocardial Fibrosis, and Beta-Blocking Drugs. This can eventually lead to cerebral anoxia and death.

Definitions for this page
Anoxia is a condition in which certain tissues of the body receive inadequate amounts of oxygen.

Homœopathic Remedies include *Helleborus* and *Kali brom.*

THE HOLISTIC PERSPECTIVE

It is easy to become anxious about treating heart disorders. Coronary heart disease is the number one killer in the UK. From a holistic perspective we need to be aware that the heart isn't only a pump, it can be seen as the seat of human emotions and, as a consequence, it is the place where we identify our feelings and often our response to the world. Any pathology with the heart may be a response to a stressor in the world around us. As holistic practitioners it will not do to treat heart pathology in isolation. What are the aetiological factors on a mental & emotional level that has lead this person to develop their pathology?

The heart occupies a unique position in our society and this is reflected in our language – people are warm hearted, big hearted, stony hearted. In grief our hearts break and in excitement they miss a beat. There is also a societal fear of heart disease, which can cause anxiety and worry, that impacts on the efficiency of the heart and thus the prophecy is fulfilled.

Don't forget that when you are treating your patients for chest pain there is only roughly 50% chance that the pain is caused by a disorder of the heart. Check carefully for the other possibilities, some of these are shown below.

Condition	Characteristics
Angina pectoris	Occurs during exertion. Radiating pain. Temporary.
Myocardial Infarction	Occurs at rest. Sweating. Nausea and vomiting.
Tracheitis	(Inflamed trachea) Cough. Scratchy pain. Localised.
Pleurisy	Local pain, peripheral, sharp and worse on inspiration.
Hiatus hernia	Burning pain, reflux after meals. Worse lying down.
Herpes Zoster	Well ... a rash ... obviously.
Bronchial cancer	Smoker, cough, weight loss, sharp pain.
Osteoarthritis	Age. Poor posture. Recurrence in certain positions.
Osteoporosis	Age. Kyphosis. Worse movement.
Referred pains	From peptic ulcer, hepatitis, cholecystitis (inflamed gallbladder), etc.

CONVENTIONAL TREATMENT

In the main, people suffering with heart diseases are frequently examined quite minutely and (as a consequence?) are found to have more than one thing wrong with them. Naturally this means that they are likely to receive more than one type of medication. Most of your patients with pathology in this area will be on a couple (or more) types of medication, and may have been given dire warnings about the consequences of stopping their pills. Wonderful.

Included amongst the options available to modern medicine in this area are drugs which affect the rate and rhythm of the heart, including anti-arryhthmics, beta-blockers, and digoxin. Other pills are available which affect the diameter of the blood vessels; either dilating them to improve blood flow, and reduce blood pressure (vasodilators) or to constrict them (vasoconstrictors). There are also a range of other medicines that can reduce blood volume, reduce fat levels, alter clotting ability, increase water excretion (diuretics), reduce cholesterol levels, reduce clotting and so on and so on.

Below are a few of the more common prescriptions likely to be seen:

DIGITALIS

This is a drug used in cases of atrial fibrillation – where the heart is beating too fast and/or slightly irregularly. It strengthens the heart muscle and reduces the flow of electrical impulses in the heart (which is a good thing if they are too frequent). There are (broadly) only two types of digitalis drug; digitoxin and digoxin; in general digoxin is preferred because it is shorter acting and easier to adjust to obtain the right therapeutic dose.

Digoxin is removed from the body via the kidneys and Digitoxin via the liver. Both are poisonous in high doses, so impairments of either the liver or kidneys will determine the most appropriate choice.

SIDE EFFECTS

Drowsiness, headache, loss of appetite, nausea, stomach upset or vomiting are the 'minor effects' and should disappear as the patient adjusts to the medication. Major side effects include bad dreams, blurred vision, breast enlargement (in both sexes), confusion, depression, disorientation, hallucinations, muscle weakness, palpitations, or tingling sensations.

BETA BLOCKERS

One of the most common beta-blockers in the UK is Propranolol. Propranolol (and other beta-adrenergic blocking agents, such as Inderal, Inderal LA, Atenolol, Nadolol and Betaxolol) is used to treat high blood pressure, angina pectoris, and irregular heartbeat. It works by controlling nerve impulses along certain nerve pathways. It is also used conventionally in preventing migraine headaches and preventing additional heart attacks in patients.

It is important to know that beta-blockers do not 'cure' high blood pressure; they only control the condition as long as they are taken.

SIDE EFFECTS

Minor side effects include: Anxiety, constipation, decreased sexual ability, diarrhoea, difficulty in sleeping, drowsiness, dryness of the eyes, mouth, and skin, headache, nausea, nervousness, stomach discomfort, tiredness or weakness. These side effects are expected to disappear as the patient adjusts to the medicine.

Major ones are: breathing difficulty or wheezing, cold hands or feet (due to decreased blood circulation to skin, fingers, and toes), confusion, depression, dizziness, hair loss, hallucinations, light-headedness, nightmares, numbness or tingling of the fingers or toes, rapid weight gain (three to five pounds within a week), reduced alertness, swelling, sore throat and fever, skin rash, or unusual bleeding or bruising.

Propranolol is one of the medicines that interact with a number of other drugs. Here are a few of the more interesting ones (really, this is just a few, I haven't listed them all):

- Indomethacin, aspirin, or other salicylates lessen the blood-pressure-lowering effects of beta-blockers.
- Cimetidine and oral contraceptives can increase the blood concentrations of Propranolol, which can result in greater side effects.
- Barbiturates, alcohol, and rifampin can increase the breakdown of Propranolol in the body, which can lead to a decrease in its effectiveness.
- Beta-blockers can also interact with insulin or oral antidiabetic agents, raising or lowering blood sugar levels or masking the symptoms of low blood sugar.
- The action of beta-blockers may be excessively increased if they are used with Chlorpromazine, Frusemide, or Hydralazine.

That's enough of the side effects; save to say that beta-blockers have the physical effect of reducing the peaks and troughs of the cardiac system. That's to say that the patient doesn't get too up or too down within normal limits. In my experience this physical effect is mirrored in the emotions of the patient. They will often find themselves experiencing neither the ups nor the downs of life. Lovely as this might be for a couple of weeks it can be wearing after a time. It also tends to 'mask' the emotional life, or as we might say, suppress it.

VASODILATORS

Vasodilators enlarge, or dilate, small blood vessels. These drugs are taken mostly to treat narrowing of the coronary arteries, the vessels that carry blood to the heart. Drugs used to enlarge these arteries are called coronary vasodilators. Doctors prescribe them for people with such severe narrowing of the coronary arteries that they suffer chest pains while walking or exercising in some other way.

The vasodilators are classed as nitrates, calcium channel blockers, sympatholytics and angiotensin-converting enzyme (ACE) inhibitors. The table below shows how each functions.

The most common and worrying side effect of these drugs is that blood pressure may fall too low, so they tend not to be prescribed for people with unstable BP, and need to be monitored.

Drug Type	Action	Examples of drug type
Nitrates	Widen the vessel by relaxing muscles surrounding the blood vessel.	Glyceryl trinitrate (TNT.)
Calcium Channel blockers	Similarly inhibit muscle contraction.	Amlodipine, Diltiazem, Felodipine.
Sympatholytics	Interfere with the nerve impulses that govern the contraction of blood vessels.	Doxazoin, Indoramin, Prazosin, Terazosin.
ACE Inhibitors	Block an enzyme in the blood which is responsible for producing angiotensin II – a vasoconstrictor.	Captopril, Quinapril, Enalapril.

DIURETICS

Finally in terms of drugs, diuretics are commonly used in the treatment of heart disorders. They increase the output of urine. The reason for increasing the flow of urine is to decrease the amount of water in the body and consequently a smaller volume of blood is circulating in the body. Thus it is easier for the heart to function. The most common side effect is a sudden reduction in potassium levels (because it's all been eliminated in the urine). This can manifest in confusion, weakness and (ironically) abnormal heart rhythms. Patients will usually be given potassium supplements with a diuretic, which minimises this problem. Common diuretics include: Bumentanide, Frusemide, Traimterene, Bendrofluazide and Metolazone.

HOMŒOPATHIC TREATMENT

CRATAEGUS OXYACANTHA

This is a remedy that has been of proven value in a range of heart conditions. Indeed it can be used as a 'heart tonic', either alone or in combination (often with *China* and *Cactus*, known as *C-C-C*) usually as a mother tincture. It can be administered as drops in water, customarily between 5 and 30 drops daily. In my experience it is a priceless tincture and is very gentle. The only downside with such gentle treatment is that it can be slow. Patients often need to take it for 3 to 6 months, or even longer, to really reap the benefit. It has been used with success for a number of heart problems including:

- Non – specific heart murmurs
- High blood pressure
- Enlarged heart
- Weakness of the heart valves
- Palpitations
- High pulse rate

One of the benefits of this kind of gentle approach is that the patient doesn't have to change their conventional medication; just give the tincture as an addition to strengthen the heart. Then, as the situation improves, the patient can negotiate with their doctor to reduce their medication. It has also been used with a tissue salt to augment its effect, most commonly *Natrum mur.*

CRATAEGUS

This is not well represented either in Materia Medicas or Repertories. Nonetheless there are many remedies whose reputation rests on their clinical efficacy rather than mountains of literature (including *Calendula* and *Echinacea*). The limited mental picture includes irritability, confusion, and a hurried feeling, but patients with none of these 'mind symptoms' have been helped enormously by this remedy.

DIGITALIS

In the past *Digitalis* was used as a remedy for gonorrhoea, and it can often be useful if there are concomitant (male) genito-urinary problems alongside the heart condition. So where a patient has a heart condition and prostate problems, or impotency, or dribbling of urine, this remedy is particularly well indicated.

There are three main indications for the use of this remedy, they are:

- Weakness of the pulse, or irregularity of the pulse, and (most importantly) slow pulse
- Pain, soreness, or enlargement of the liver
- White stools

It is (as you might guess) a good remedy for elderly men with a heart condition – especially if they have raised blood pressure.

A note of warning: Digitalis is still used in a few conventional medicines for heart conditions, and it would be inadvisable to use the homœopathic version concurrently.

OTHER HEART REMEDIES

There are, of course, any number of remedies that will be indicated in heart conditions. As usual a well-taken case should lead to both specific and constitutional solutions. Just as a quick aide-memoir here are half a dozen of the more 'obvious' choices…this is, of necessity, greatly simplified.

AURUM MET

Heart conditions with associated depression, palpitations, high blood pressure, arteriosclerosis, pain at night behind the sternum.

ACONITE

Acute heart conditions which come on suddenly and cause the patient to fear for their life. Anxiety, restlessness, fear, Tachycardia (increase in heart rate), tingling in the fingers and full, hard pulse.

ARNICA

Heart attack following trauma, or unusual exertions, Angina attacks, pains in the left elbow. Feebleness of the pulse, oedema around the heart and distressing breathlessness.

ARSENICUM

Palpitations with pain, breathlessness, faintness and fear. Rapid pulse in the morning. Angina with pain in the neck.

LACHESIS

Palpitations and constriction. Irregular heartbeat and cyanosis. Lachesis has profound prostration and a strong dislike of tight clothing. There is also a tendency to either sleep into an attack or sleep creates an aggravation of the condition.

CACTUS

Cardiac incompetence. The heart feels constricted as if by an 'iron band'. Violent palpitations, which are worse lying on the left side. Angina, with a cold, cold sweat and a feeling of great suffocation.

Pathology of the circulation

We have something in the order of 75,000 miles of blood vessels in the body, so it's hardly surprising that there are the odd problem or two…

THE CIRCULATION

ATHEROMA & ATHEROSCLEROSIS

Starting with the 'A's. Atheroma is degeneration of the walls of the arteries due to the formation of fatty plaques and scar tissue. Obviously this is going to limit the flow of the blood and predispose the patient to thrombosis (a change of the blood from liquid to solid, thus forming clots, as we've said earlier). Atheroma is common to us in the Western world and is attributed to a diet rich in animal fats and refined sugar. Not to mention our massive consumption of cigarettes. Other contributory factors may include obesity, a lack of exercise and of course high blood pressure.

Atheroma may be completely symptom-less until later life when it can be a contributory factor in a number of diseases including:

- Angina Pectoris
- Heart Attack

- Strokes
- Gangrene

Conventional treatment is really aimed at prevention, although in severe cases of Atheroma it is possible to bypass the affected area. The difference between Atheroma and Atherosclerosis is that the former is the name of the condition and the latter of the disease. To all intents and purposes they are pretty much interchangeable.

Remedies to consider for this condition include:

Remedy	Characteristics
Lachesis	Cyanosis, irregular heart beat, constriction and anxiety. < after sleep, sleeps into aggravation. > discharges.
Vanadium	Wasting, degeneration of the arteries, sensation as if the heart were compressed, as if the blood has no room in the aorta. Pressure on the whole chest, fatty heart.

HARDENED ARTERIES

This is to some degree a natural process – as we age there is an increasing deposit of calcium in the artery and this can lead to hardening, remedies to consider include:

Remedy	Characteristics
Aurum mur	Restlessness, > cold washing and cold weather. < ascending stairs, Warmth. Throws off bedclothes.
Badiaga	> heat, warm room. < cold air, pressure, touch, < stormy weather.

ANEURYSMS

These are swellings in the wall of an artery. They can be caused by degenerative diseases or syphilitic infection (so check out the possible miasmatic connection here), which damages the muscular coat of the vessel. These may also be due to a congenital defect (although once again we can be quite confident about the miasm). They can occur in any large artery. The symptoms are severe chest pain, described as a tearing pain often extending to the back, accompanied by shock (these can be misdiagnosed as myocardial infarction).

Aneurysms can also occur in the abdomen and between an artery and a vein (arteriovenous aneurysm). If the connection is large the 'short circuiting' of the blood can produce heart failure. There is also the possibility of aneurysm in the brain (a congenital disorder in all likelihood), which, if it bursts, can cause subarachnoid haemorrhage.

Homœopathic remedies for aneurysms include:

Remedy	Area affected	Characteristics
Calc carb	Large arteries	Chest very sensitive to touch or pressure.
Cuprum met	Large arteries	H/O Angina. Slow pulse, fatty degeneration.
Bartya mur	Abdomen	Gone feeling at epigastrium, retching and vomiting.
Secale	Abdomen	<heat, warm covering, > cold, uncovering.
Calendula	Aorta	< damp, heavy, cloudy weather.
Spongia	Aorta	< ascending, wind, before midnight. > descending, lying with head low.
Carbo veg	Heart	< evening, night, open air, > fanning, eructation, cold.

RAYNAUD'S DISEASE

Raynaud's Disease and Raynaud's Phenomenon are vascular disorders. These disorders have spasms of arterioles (that's a small branch of the artery) occurring especially in the fingers and toes and occasionally in other acral (extremity) parts of the body such as the nose and tongue. The intermittent attacks of pallor or cyanosis of the digits may be precipitated by exposure to cold or by emotional upsets. It may be either idiopathic (idiopathic means a disease whose cause is 'spontaneous' or unknown) or secondary to other conditions. Raynaud's Disease is usually benign, causing only mild discomfort and progressing very slightly over the years. In some cases, however, there is a rapid progression of the disorder, which may result in sclerodactyly (loss of subcutaneous tissue) or small painful ulcers may appear on the tips of the affected digits.

SIGNS AND SYMPTOMS

Attacks of both Raynaud's Disease and Phenomenon occur more frequently in cold rather than hot weather. Symptoms associated with Raynaud's Disease may include a feeling of numbness and coldness of the toes or fingers. Only one or two fingertips may be involved early in the course of the disease. As the disorder progresses, all the fingers down to the palm may be affected, although the thumbs are rarely involved.

RAYNAUD'S PHENOMENON

This is the same set of symptoms but is associated with an external cause such as systemic lupus.

Patients may experience sensory changes such as an aching pain, tingling feeling, or throbbing in the afflicted digits. There may be the sensation of tightness or pins and needles.

Onset is usually in the first or second decade of life. The vasospasm attacks may last from minutes to hours, but are rarely severe enough to result in gross tissue loss.

The colour changes in Raynaud's phenomenon may be either triphasic (pallor, cyanosis, and redness followed by reactive hyperaemia – the term hyperaemia denotes excess blood) or biphasic (cyanosis followed by reactive hyperaemia). Rewarming the affected digits results in a return to normal colour and sensation.

HOMŒOPATHIC TREATMENT

Raynaud's Disease is a condition that is seen quite frequently in homœopathic clinics (this may be a reflection of patient dissatisfaction with the conventional approach), and experience shows that homœopathy can be effective in relief or removal of symptoms.

Remedies to consider include *Agaricus, Hepar sulph, Rhus tox, Sepia,* and *Silica.*

VARICOSE VEIN

This is a dilated and often tortuous vein. If a vein becomes permanently dilated it is called a varicose vein. This occurs because the valves in the vein no longer function properly or because blood volume in the vein increases; usually both conditions occur together and are interrelated. Theoretically any vein can develop varicosities, but certain veins are more likely to.

When veins in the submucous membranes of the rectum dilate, haemorrhoids, or piles, result. These may be painful and may bleed. Treatment can vary but often surgery is necessary. When the spermatic veins in the scrotum dilate, a Variocele results. This commonly occurs on the left side and may enlarge, become annoying or painful, and require surgery.

The most common varicose veins are the superficial leg veins. These become rather prominent and readily visible. In addition to being a bluish colour, they may cause ankle oedema and skin ulcerations.

Venous thromboses (blood clots), which are tender and painful, may develop and may break off and become obstructions elsewhere, particularly in the pulmonary arterioles.

Conventionally simple superficial varicose leg veins are treated by applying pressure all along them with an elastic stocking, by sclerosing them with a chemical solution, or by removing them surgically. In these latter instances, because the blood usually carried in them is diverted to the deep leg veins, the deep veins must be functioning normally.

Homœopathically it is important to (as ever) examine the underlying cause of varicose veins and attend to that. However, appropriate remedies may include *Arnica, Carbo veg Hamamelis, Fluoric acid* and *Sepia.*

DEEP VEIN THROMBOSIS

This is where the blood clots in one of the deep veins of the calf or the pelvis, often because the flow has become rather sluggish, dehydrated or because of trauma. These events occur most commonly after childbirth, abdominal surgery and heart attacks. The blood may also clot because of abnormal proteins present in certain cancers or due to drugs (notably the pill) containing oestrogens.

Symptoms usually include some aching in the calf and a little swelling, possibly with slight fever, although often there are no symptoms.

The most hazardous consequence of DVT is that a piece will break off and travel to the inferior vena cava as an embolism and from there to the lungs. Here it can block the arteriole where it rests with the threat of Ischaemia and possible infarction of a portion of the lung.

Pulmonary embolism is one of the main causes of sudden death after an operation and is most likely to happen at one-week post-operative.

The best treatment from a homœopathic point of view is prophylactically prior to operations, possibly with a vein organ remedy such as *Cascarilla* or one of the circulatory remedies outlined in the heart section.

HEADACHES (SEE PAGE 28)

While many are be cardiovascular in origin they are all covered under the Musculoskeletal System.

FURTHER READING

Jan Scholten **Homœopathy and the Elements**
Published by Stichting Alonissos
Email: alonnissos@tip.nl *(No ISBN Number)*

Dr. Kailash Narayan Mathur **Principles of Prescribing**
B Jain Publishers
ISBN 81-7021-454-8

A Blackwood **Diseases of the Heart**
B Jain Publishers
ISBN 81-7021-213-8

E Balakrishan **Cardiovascular Diseases and Homœopathic Treatment**
B Jain Publishers
ISBN 81-8056-470-3

F Burnoville **Remedies of Circulatory and Respiratory System**
B Jain Publishers
ISBN :81-7021-655-9

NOTES

NOTES

CONTENTS

THE RESPIRATORY SYSTEM

OVERVIEW

The respiratory tract, where external respiration occurs, starts at the nose and mouth. It then extends to the trachea (windpipe) from the neck into the thorax, where it divides into right and left main bronchi, which enter the right and left lungs, breaking up as they do so into smaller bronchi and bronchioles and ending in small air sacs called alveoli, where the exchange of gases occurs.

The lungs are divided into right and left; the left is the smaller of the two as that space also accommodates the heart.

The surface area of the lungs in an adult is around 140 square metres – roughly the size of a tennis court.

The respiratory tract, from the nose right through to the smallest parts of the lungs, is lined by a layer of sticky mucus, secreted by the epithelium assisted by small ducted glands. This is one of the many protective systems the body uses to shield this delicate organ from the external environment that is brought into the body with every breath. Particles that hit the sidewall of the tract are trapped in the mucus. Once the particles have been 'trapped' by the mucus they have to be removed, as indeed does the mucus. This is carried out by cilia on the epithelial cells that move the mucus continually up or down the tract towards the nose and mouth. The mucus and its trapped particles are then swallowed.

The lungs also warm the air (or cool it as appropriate) – the length of the respiratory tract helps in both bringing the air to the right temperature and humidity. The entry of food and drink into the larynx is prevented by the structure of the larynx and by the fact that swallowing is quite a complex act.

To recap then, the functions of the respiratory system are:

- To allow chemical changes – to acquire oxygen and to eliminate carbon dioxide.
- To clean the air (or more accurately to filter it).
- Warm or cool the air as appropriate.

Just as it is helpful sometimes to view the heart as two organs (left and right) so it can be useful to see that there are two types of respiration – external and internal.

- External respiration is what we normally view as respiration; it is where gases are exchanged between the lungs and the blood…the blood 'gains' oxygen.
- Internal respiration is the end result (the 'point') of respiration wherein gases are exchanged between the blood and the cells of the body…the cells gain oxygen, the blood removes CO_2.

It is possible to view the internal respiratory process as one whose efficiency is increased by appropriate homœopathy (as indeed can any bodily process). It is also feasible that improved efficiency at the cellular exchange level will result in the cells being better resourced (with oxygen) and will also aid the release of any toxins stored at the cellular level.

This offers one explanation of the homœopathic aggravation and of Hering's Law that 'old' diseases reoccur. If the detritus of old diseases are stored at the cellular level they may be released by improved internal respiration and thus briefly reawaken old diseases.

SINUSITIS

The sinuses are air cavities within the bones of the face or skull. Sinusitis therefore is an inflammation of one or more of these 'air spaces'. The spaces are lined by mucus and it is common that infection spreads from the nose, with which the cavities communicate. The typical symptoms include:

- Pain across the nose
- A feeling of obstruction
- Catarrh and mucus
- Often occurs at the end of a cold
- Pressure at the root of the nose
- A sensation of toothache in the head
- Headache < stooping
- Voice changes

CONVENTIONAL TREATMENT

This will often focus on clearing any infection. However, in extreme and persistent cases, treatment may require the affected sinus to be washed out or drained by a surgical operation.

HOMŒOPATHIC TREATMENT

From a homœopathic perspective there are two other common symptoms that can help to guide to a remedy. Yellow/green muco-pus is not an untypical symptom and *Natrum sulph* can often be a great help. If the mucus is particularly thick and difficult to expel, then *Kali bic* is frequently a brilliant remedy. *Kali bic* is usually < in the morning and < on stooping.

Indeed the esteemed George Vithoulkas says for sinusitis use *Kali bic* unless there is something better indicated. It is also usually < cold damp weather > warm bed. *Silica* has a similar picture to *Kali bic*, but with no discharge.

SORE THROATS

Sore throats are often the result of an infection; these include:

- Viral infections – often pharyngitis or laryngitis
- Bacterial infections

- Strep throat
- Respiratory or upper respiratory tract infection

It might be helpful to know that pharyngitis is a viral infection that irritates the nerve in the throat (or the face) and laryngitis is also a viral infection, tubercular in nature and is more liable to be an allergic response to inhalation of toxins, poisons, fumes, etc.

CONVENTIONAL TREATMENT

This is inevitably going to concentrate on elimination of the infection, and palliative treatment to soothe the throat.

It is worth noting however, that there are a number of other possible causes of sore throats, and that a persistent or debilitating sore throat should be cause for concern. Here are some of the other possible causes of sore throat:

- Gingivitis
- Hand, foot and mouth disease
- Scarlet fever
- Measles
- Gonorrhoea
- Chickenpox

Space concerns prohibit looking at each of these conditions (or indeed listing all the possible causes of sore throat). The important point is that we should not consider a sore throat as an insignificant condition.

Additionally, with any sore throats there are two things to look out for:

1) If it is a very long-standing infection is there a maintaining cause?
2) Changes in the voice. Any sudden changes in the voice may be of concern and could indicate a tumour.
3) Homœopathic treatment

Given the caveats about treating sore throats lightly, there are a few remedies that have proven themselves time and again to be of great help. Among those to consider are *Phosphorus* and *Rumex* – these may be thought of as '1st choice' remedies.

Second choices would include: *Carbo veg*..... below par, colds do not clear, voice becomes husky especially in the evenings, exhausting cough...like whooping cough, red in the face, larynx raw and tender to the touch.

Drosera.... cough comes on after eating or drinking.

ADJUNCTIVE ADVICE

It would be good to reduce smoking if that is a factor. Also many practitioners like to use linctus, which soothes the throat. A good homœopathic pharmacy will stock linctus containing one or more remedies (possibly *Bryonia*).

Of course a sore throat is often a concomitant symptom to coughs and colds, if that is the case then the next section may be of some help.

CROUP, COUGHS & COLDS

This is likely to be a huge part of any practice, and consequently I have given over quite a bit of space to it. Most practitioners find that any work they put in to learning how to deal with coughs and colds is well worth it. Success with these common conditions can be the wellspring of a busy practice.

COUGHS AND CROUP

In much of the older homœopathic literature it is unclear what the difference is between a cough and croup. Croup is still a term used these days; it simply means that there is a partial obstruction caused by a swelling of the larynx (the small cup-shaped section just above the trachea). It is most commonly used when referring to a hollow resonating cough in young children.

Croup therefore can obstruct the airway, it is most common amongst children and the usual symptoms include a deep barking cough, and anxiety. Other symptoms include:

- Harshness and/or difficulty in breathing
- A rising pulse rate
- Restlessness
- Cyanosis

CONVENTIONAL TREATMENT

The symptoms of croup can be a bit scary, both for the child and the parents. Conventional treatment aims to reduce these symptoms by mild sedation and humidification. In very severe cases the obstruction to breathing is considered dangerous and surgery may be needed (a tracheostomy, commonly).

It is worth being aware that croup may be a precursor to tonsillitis.

HOMŒOPATHIC TREATMENT

As the patient and their parents are likely to be alarmed by the symptoms, homœopathic treatment should be swift and accurate. If it hasn't already been advised, then humidification will help (a hot steamy bath maybe).

THE MOST COMMON CROUP REMEDIES.

Remedy	Characteristics
Spongia	Deep and hoarse barking cough, anxiety.
Belladonna	Fever, red face, dry skin and mouth.
Antimonium tart	Rattling sounds in the chest, expectoration difficult.
Iodum	Wheezing, sawing respiration, child grabs their throat.
Hepar Sulph	Croup develops after midnight.

THE COMMON COLD

It's hardly worth looking at any of the cough literature without acknowledging that, in practice, you will frequently be dealing with a cough and a cold concurrently.

There is some dispute amongst homœopaths as to whether it is advisable to treat colds or whether to see them as beneficial; in that the body is eliminating toxins, and the elimination may be a positive reaction for the patient. I leave this knotty philosophical argument to you to sort out.

However, if you do see a patient with more than two or three colds per month, it's a fairly safe bet that something is wrong. Along with a well-chosen constitutional remedy you should also consider *Tuberculinum*.

If you do treat colds (usually your own in my experience) then the stand-by remedies are those shown on the table below. It's worth bearing in mind that colds are not easy to treat and you are unlikely to impress with miracle cures. The problems are twofold; the symptom picture changes so quickly and a cold is often nature's way of saying "have a week off and lie down with hot water bottles and take it easy". So often nothing will work without time off from the hurly burly of everyday life.

HOMŒOPATHIC TREATMENT

The table overleaf shows some (but nothing like all) of the remedies that you could think of for the common cold with or without the accompanying cough.

REMEDIES FOR THE COMMON COLD

Remedy	Comments
Gelsemium	Drowsy, droopy, dizzy and weak.
Eupatorium Perf	Aching, painful to move. Catarrh.
Aconite	Given early may forestall the cold.
Arsenicum	Watery catarrh and sore nostrils.
Pulsatilla	Intermittent, thick catarrh, no thirst, > outside.

CHILDREN

Right. So let's have a look at the presentation of the cough, as it will be seen in the more 'typical' children's constitutional cases. In other words, if we assume (or acknowledge) that the most frequently needed children's remedies are:

Calc carb	Lycopodium	Medorrhinum
Silica	Phosphorus	Sulphur
Natrum mur	Pulsatilla	Tuberculinum

- then how would you expect to see respiratory disease in general and coughs in particular manifest in these children? The following offer indications for these most common remedies. Of course this is not a comprehensive guide either to the condition or the remedies, but sometimes a 'quick guide' can be of more immediate use than fulsome information.

CALCAREA CARBONICA

Most respiratory infections result in a cough, as do any allergic responses. The cough is dry at night, but loose in the morning. In young children the cough may be accompanied by high fever. Tiredness, irritability, and the typical hot head with cold extremities.

Expectoration can be thick, yellow, and sometimes smells foul. These are tickling coughs.

< cold, < wet, < wind. Cold, damp feet.

LYCOPODIUM

Lycopodium children are prone to coughs with bronchitis or pneumonia. Often after an acute infection, a lingering cough will remain.

This is the cough that will keep the child up at night (and they are the sort of child who will keep the parents up too.) It is aggravated at night, when lying down. There can be rattling in the chest when breathing, and the keynote flaring of the nostrils may be seen. Most colds will progress to a cough and possibly bronchitis.

MEDORRHINUM

These children are prone to asthma anyway and may have an accompanying, lingering cough. Both will be aggravated by damp cold weather, notably in the spring

They are better for lying down and may, when they start to cough, throw themselves on the bed burying their head in the pillow. In this position they may also find it easier to sleep.

The cough can be a deep rattling one. No matter how hard they try they can't dislodge the mucus. So they are left with a constant, dry cough. Expectoration (if they can do it) will be green/yellow and clumpy.

NATRUM MURIATICUM

The cough of Natrum mur may precede asthma. It begins with a dry, hollow cough that sounds like a dog's bark. Following this comes shortness of breath, and a tightening of the chest.

Both the cough and the asthma can be attributed to emotional aetiologies.

There can be allergic coughs (< dust, autumn, exertion, evening,) again with the possibility of an emotional aetiology.

PHOSPHORUS

The lungs are one of the main areas of action in this remedy – so it's inevitably a big cough remedy. From quite a young age, any cold quickly descends to the lungs and causes coughs and bronchitis.

The coughs are < cold air and lying on the left.

Also < eating, drinking and talking.

The cough is worse in the morning, gets better through the day and is then becomes worse from sundown to midnight.

The cough can be painful and children can hold onto their breath, because they know that when they breathe in they cough and when they cough it really hurts.

PULSATILLA

This is another remedy that has an affinity for the lungs with frequent problems, both acute and chronic.

It is one of the remedies for croup where it commences with a dry cough, < at night and with a sensation as if the throat were closing down at the larynx. Naturally enough this is worse when the child goes to sleep (whilst lying down) and can also be accompanied by retching and/or vomiting.

The cough may have a dry tickle in the throat which is < warmth, overheating and exertion. The cough will eventually become productive creating a thick, yellow discharge. This is 'bland' and easily dislodged.

One of the keynotes of the cough is that it is dry during the day and night, then loose and 'wet' on waking (with concomitant expectoration.) Pulsatilla shares this keynote with Calcarea carbonica.

Pulsatilla is another of the remedies that can be allergic to the environment, so the child may develop a cough in response to pollen, house dust, etc.

SULPHUR

Sulphur has a whole host of lung and respiratory system problems (in common with every other system too, it has to be said.) There may be a history of colds, coughs, asthma, bronchitis and so forth, often associated with skin eruptions. The eruption may alternate with the cough or precede it. The cough is exhausting, causing breathing difficulties and perspiration on the face – in acute attacks they may need Arsenicum album, with Sulphur as a constitutional preventative.

Coughs and asthma are triggered by household allergies, especially exposure to mould or cats.

The cough is hard, dry and hacking, finally yielding a white or yellow expectoration. It is < lying on the back, < warm rooms and < getting warm at night. > open air. They feel suffocated and want the doors and windows open.

TUBERCULINUM

Lung problems can begin at birth for the Tuberculinum children and most catch colds frequently. These colds settle into a persistent cough and the history should reveal diseases such as bronchitis, whooping cough, croup and so on. They are < damp, smoke and pollution generally. The cough is dry and worse at night, they can even cough during their sleep. At night there is no expectoration but in the morning, if it comes, it will be thick, yellow and pus-like. It tastes sweet or salty. Tubercular children have the chronic cough as well as acute episodes, and they complain of a tickle at the back of the throat. Because the lungs are so weak they are slow to recuperate and may only just recover when the next bout strikes. The cough is 'always there' it simply deteriorates during acute episodes. There is often an aetiology of the cough following exposure to cold air and/or a fever.

Finally here is (another) table showing the other leading contenders for the award of 'Remedy Most Likely To Fix The Cold'. As ever in homœopathy there can be any number of remedies that may work, but these, added to those on the previous pages will cover 90% of colds.

Remedy	Comments	Modalities
Aconite	Constant, short, dry cough. Feels suffocated. Hoarse, dry, loud, ringing cough. Cough wakes from sleep. Anxiety and fear. Restlessness.	Worse at night. Comes on suddenly. Follows cold, dry winds.
Belladonna	Dry cough from dryness of larynx. Cough with redness in throat. Tickling, burning and scraping sensation. Cough as if head would burst. Child cries before the cough. Spasmodic, barking and short cough.	< touch, jar, noise,draught. < afternoon, lying down.
Bryonia	Hard dry cough with sore chest. Cough with stitches in the chest and headache- as if head would 'fly to pieces.' Irritable. Wants to be left alone. Thirsty.	< night, eating and drinking. < entering a warm room. < taking deep breaths. < east winds. < movement, pressure.

Remedy	Comments	Modalities
Nux vomica	Dry teasing cough. Cold which travels to the chest. Fever. Cannot move without feeling cold. Spasms and retching. Cough causes headache. Acute laryngitis. Whooping cough. Hypersensitive.	< cold, dry and windy.
Hepar sulph	Cough when any part of the body becomes uncovered. Suffocative coughing spells. Croup from cold, dry wind.	<cold, dry weather. > warm moist weather. < breathing cold air. < putting hand out of bed.
Causticum	Dryness, soreness, rawness. Hoarseness, aphonia. Hard cough-racks the whole chest. With each cough a drop of urine escapes.	> ice cold water
Spongia	Cough sounds like a saw driven through a board. Wakes with suffocation, anxiety and alarm. Tough mucus – has to be swallowed.	< talking, reading, singing. < Swallowing. < lying with head low.
Rhus tox	Dry, teasing cough from tickling in bronchia. Nocturnal cough. Taste of blood (but no blood visible.) Cough during sleep.	< uncovering < cold, wet weather. < uncovering. Restless.
Drosera	Crawling in larynx which provokes cough. Spasm, retching and vomiting. Dyspnoea with cough. Hoarseness. Whooping cough.	< night.
Rumex	Cough on changing rooms – from breathing cold air. Covers mouth up. Tough stringy mucus. Dyspnoea.	<going from warm to cold. Sensitive to open air.
Arsenicum	Wheezing with cough. Cannot breathe fully. Cough with asthma. Prostration and debility. Burning pains.	< after midnight-1 a.m.

BRONCHITIS

This can be an acute or a chronic condition. Acutely, it is an upper respiratory tract infection with the following symptoms:

- Irritating dry cough
- Fever
- Tightness of the chest
- Expectoration of mucus/pus/both

Chronically bronchitis is related to working in a poor environment (or living in one), or smoking or pollution in the environment. The chronic condition has symptoms of:

- Thick green pus
- Raised temperature
- Tightness of the chest, especially in the morning

Good advice is to stay away from the irritant (which has proved particularly difficult for some smokers of course), stay warm and exercise.

BRONCHITIS IN CHILDREN

Bronchitis is particularly distressing for children in acute attacks (and for the parents), the typical picture is of:

- Increased mucus production
- Rales (a wheezing sound) on the chest
- Increase in temperature
- Very distressing cough

CONVENTIONAL TREATMENT – CHILDREN AND ADULTS

Conventionally this disease is thought to be caused by a viral infection that usually resolves itself within a few days. Secondary infections are treated with antibiotics and usually respond quite quickly. In cases of some distress, taking painkillers may be suggested. Most health professionals will emphasise the importance of giving up smoking.

MEDICATION

It is likely that patients who suffer from bronchitis will be on some form of conventional medication. A drug used to reduce the stickiness and viscosity of mucus can be used (for example Acetylcysteine). These are known as a mucolytics, and are used for freeing sputum in bronchitis. Another choice may be a bronchodilator such as Rimiterol or Salbutamol.

HOMŒOPATHIC TREATMENT

Ipecac is a good remedy of first choice – indicated by constant, violent coughing…with every breath, and a sense of tightness in the chest.

If the patient is more obviously ill, has a lot of wheezing, is slightly cyanosed and has a coated tongue then *Antimonium tart* may be invaluable.

It is fairly common in adults to see an acute recurrence every winter of what is essentially a chronic condition ("every year I get an attack of bronchitis"), in this scenario *Antimonium carb* is a good remedy. There are many, many remedies that may be of use in bronchitis. As ever, there is a necessity for good case taking.

PNEUMONIA

This is a bacterial or viral inflammatory infection of the lungs, in which the alveoli (the air sacs) fill up with pus. This obviously means that air is excluded from the lungs to some degree, and in severe cases part of the lung can become solid with the following symptoms:

- Presence of pneumococcus
- High temperature
- Dry fever
- Chest pain
- Flushing
- Dry cough…that becomes loose and productive
- Cold sores – interestingly

CONVENTIONAL TREATMENT

The bacteria that usually cause pneumonia are sensitive to antibiotics, and thus conventional treatment can be rapid and effective.

HOMŒOPATHIC TREATMENT

Because conventional treatment is quick, generally effective, and aimed at swiftly reducing discomfort, homœopathic intervention needs to be equally successful. So it is imperative to gather all the necessary information and make an impact on the disease in a short time. Any of the remedies that have an affinity to the respiratory system may be appropriate. The following table shows two such possibilities.

Remedy	Characteristics
Bryonia	Patients are toxic, heavy and slightly cyanotic. They dislike being disturbed and have a very painful cough with pains in the chest ++ Very thirsty. > pressure.
Phosphorus	Anxious, flushed, also thirsty, tongue not coated, dislike pressure, more alert than Bryonia.

NB Bryonia develops more slowly

TUBERCULOSIS

This disease is on the increase. Most hospitals see several cases a month. It is found largely, but not uniquely in immigrants and latterly has been 'reoccurring' in the large army of people who are sleeping rough in many cities in the UK, most commonly in elderly males. Symptoms include:

- Weight loss
- Persistent cough
- Night sweats
- "Not feeling well"
- Coughing up blood

Tuberculosis is usually caught by inhalation of bacteria that lodge in the lung; monocytes build a wall around the bacteria to prevent it spreading. This forms a capsule within which the phagocytes operate…this is primary tuberculosis.

This might be a good time to clarify our terms:

- Monocytes are a variety of white blood cell whose function is the ingestion of foreign particles.
- Phagocytes are the cells which are able to engulf and digest bacteria, protozoa and other cell debris. Phagocytes include many white blood cells and macrophages.
- Macrophages are large scavenger cells present in connective tissue and many major organs.

In primary tuberculosis there is little to notice but eventually the capsule will calcify and show as spots on an X-Ray.

Lung tissue calcification, resulting from pulmonary tuberculosis, appears as patches within the chest area of the human X ray.

When airborne sputum (expectorated phlegm) contaminated with the bacillus Mycobacterium tuberculosis is inhaled, nodular lesions, called tubercles, form in the lungs and spread through the nearest lymph node. About one-quarter of the general population is infected with the bacilla that causes tuberculosis, but most of them show no signs of the disease as long as their immune systems can keep it in check. A wonderful demonstration of the important part that susceptibility plays in our health.

Very few cases become active, and even fewer reach the potentially fatal pulmonary stage, characterised by extreme respiratory distress.

The manifestation of tuberculosis can occur anywhere in the body if the patient's circumstances change. When it spreads this is called Miliary Tuberculosis and can be fatal.

CONVENTIONAL TREATMENT

This is based on rigorous and long-term use of antibiotics – usually for at least six months. Over the past decade or so, some strains of tuberculosis have become resistant to the standard antibiotics.

HOMŒOPATHIC TREATMENT

It is unlikely that you would be called upon to treat active tuberculosis. It is anyway a notifiable disease. But as an academic exercise, the remedies to consider would include *Tuberculinum*, *Calc carb*, *Phosphorus*, *Psorinum*, *Pulsatilla*…and many, many others.

You are more likely to be in a position where you might wish to give a prophylactic for tuberculosis and certainly *Tuberculinum*, *Baccilinum*, *Calc phos*, *Phosphorus* and *Sulphur* are said to be helpful in these circumstances (see Murphy's Repertory page 445).

CANCER

The lung rarely produces primary tumours, so lung cancer is usually 'secondary'. Nonetheless cancer of the respiratory system is the third most common form (being beaten only by skin cancer and cancer of the prostate). However, cancer of the respiratory system is the most common form of death from cancer.

Lung cancer begins when epithelial cells lining the respiratory tract start to reproduce in an uncontrolled fashion. These cells invade surrounding tissue, forming a mass called a tumour and, when hardened, a carcinoma.

Cancerous cells may penetrate blood and lymph vessels, to be carried through the body until they reach a juncture through which they cannot pass. At this point, they lodge and new tumours form. Metastasis (the spreading of cancer from its original location to other parts of the body) is the disease's most destructive characteristic. From the lung, cancer can spread to the liver, bones and the brain.

Symptoms to look out for include:

Dry (unproductive) cough

- Wheezing
- Shortness of breath
- Cyanosis at the periphery

CONVENTIONAL TREATMENT

Conventional treatment is usually based on chemotherapy or radiotherapy, or a combination of the two. Both are particularly brutal responses to the disease and can have a huge impact on the patient. However, most patients with lung (or any) cancer opt to use homœopathy as a complement rather than an alternative to conventional medicine. Consequently it often falls to the homœopath to alleviate the effects of the conventional treatment as much as attempting to deal with the disease.

HOMŒOPATHIC TREATMENT

Allopathically there is often a poor diagnosis for lung cancer. Remedies that are said to have a positive effect include: *Lobelia*, *Hydrastis*, *Caladium*, *Antimonium tart*, *Morgan*.

Just for your information, if you are treating anyone who has cancer and decides to accept chemotherapy and/or radiation treatment (which as we've seen is pretty common in practice) the following remedies can be helpful in combating the side effects of those treatments:

CHEMOTHERAPY;

When on treatment give combination remedy *Cadmium sulph* 200/*Arnica* 200/ *Pyrogen* 30. When they come to the 'rest days' give *Proteus* 30. Support remedies include *Hydrastis* and *Chelidonium* in tincture. Experience has shown that these remedies can significantly reduce some of the 'side effects' of chemotherapy; notably the terrible nausea, sickness, and weakness.

RADIOTHERAPY

Give *Radium brom* and/or *Radiation combination remedy* (available from Helios Homœopathic Pharmacy).

ASTHMA

Asthma is a condition characterised by paroxysmal attacks of bronchospasm – this causes difficulty in breathing. The attacks may have no discernible cause or may be associated with a specific allergy or with stress.

CONVENTIONAL MEDICAL TREATMENT:

- Avoidance of allergens
- Medications

It is so common to see patients suffering with asthma on some form of conventional medication that it is almost universal. Consequently we need to have a close look at the likely medicines they will be using:

Inhaled beta2 agonists (e.g. Ventolin, Salbutamol). These relax the bronchial muscles and reduce the chemicals that cause inflammation. These are the 'least harmful' of the available medicaments and can be withdrawn at any time.

- Anti-inflammatories (e.g. INTAL) These drugs, called 'mast stabilisers', work by preventing the mast cells which line the bronchial tubes from releasing chemicals which make the bronchial muscles contract. Effectively therefore, this method of treatment can prevent an attack but would not be effective during an attack. Side effects of INTAL include anaphylactic shock, pneumonia, wheezing, coughing and bronchospasms (the very things which it is supposed to inhibit). Also present may be dizziness, headache, urticaria, photodermititis and vertigo.

- Steroid inhalers (e.g. Becotide). Side effects of inhaled steroids can include growth retardation in children, obesity, "moon face", thinning skin, stretch marks and easy bruising. Suppression of the immune system may also occur, this may makes otherwise benign infections have a greater impact on the system and, indeed, can cause some infections to be life threatening (notably measles, chickenpox). In adults, prolonged use of steroid inhalers may lead to reduction in bone formation, oral thrush, raised BP., muscle weakness, hyperglycaemia, water retention, insomnia, mood changes and glaucoma.

THE DISEASE

Over the past decade the incidence of diagnosed asthma has doubled. Some of this increase may be due to greater awareness and an increased 'willingness' to diagnose asthma. However some of the increase must be due to an actual growth in occurrence. Possible factors would include higher levels of pollution and stress. It is also possible that well insulated homes, double-glazing and central heating are contributory factors. In the same time frame, hospital admissions have risen five-fold for young children. In the mid-eighties the annual death rate for asthmatic related illness was running at around 2,000 per annum, whereas in the 1950's the figure was almost zero.

THE TYPICAL PICTURE

There are two aetiologies in children; which are commonly seen in practice, these are:

- Eczema which has been suppressed (or more commonly is claimed by the parent to have been 'cured').
- Vaccinations.

SIGNS & SYMPTOMS

In treating asthma it would be normal to expect the following symptoms, as they are typical of the disease:

- Alleged allergic reaction
- Difficult expiration
- < Exertion
- Periodicity
- < Stress
- Wheezing
- Tightness of the chest
- Breathlessness

NATURAL HEALING

Vitamin B6 has been shown to be of benefit to asthma sufferers as many of these patients are lacking in Pyridoxine. The recommended dose is 200mg daily. Early work suggests that asthmatics are not actually lacking in B6 but that a disturbance of the metabolism may lead them to need more of it. The typical improvements from B6 therapy would take a couple of months to occur.

Thyme baths (infusion) are supposed to have a very beneficial effect for asthmatics. These should be taken at night. Culpepper says that thyme is "a noble strengthener of the lungs, as notable as one that grows.... and is an excellent remedy for shortness of breath". Grieve (1931) says it is an "antispasmodic, tonic and carmative". Hoffman (1990) suggests that it be used in infusion for asthmatic problems. The infusions can be steamed in baths. Most of the activity of thyme is probably due to Thymol and Carvacrol, which is thought to have a potent effect on the trachea.

THE HOLISTIC PERSPECTIVE

Asthmatics, it is said, have an inability to breathe for themselves They feel stifled. The lungs are believed to be the seat of emotions, and suppression of emotions may lead to asthmatic response.

In Chinese medicine the lungs relate to grief, sorrow and sadness. As homœopaths we know this correspondence; our number one remedy for grief is probably *Ignatia*, which is also our number one remedy whose leading indication is 'sighing'.

It is also worth bearing in mind that the lungs are used to acquire oxygen – one of our main sources of energy. Consequently the work that we do with a patient's respiratory system, as well as dealing with primary pathology, will also affect the patient's energy levels. Good work will increase the energy available to the patient.

ASTHMA TREATMENT WITHOUT DRUGS

System	Advice	Dose
Avoid	Dairy products. Excessive dust/pollens.	
Supplements	B6. Vitamin C. Zinc. Vitamin E.	200mg. 500mg. 10mg. 600 IUs.
Diet	Low in sugar, dairy, animal fat, additives. High in grains and vegetables.	
Exercise	Regular gentle aerobic exercise e.g. walking, swimming.	Daily.
Herbs	Thyme, Lobelia, Coltsfoot, Ephedra.	
Homœopathy	Arsenicum, Natrum sulph, Oxygen, Medorrhinum.	30c or 200c.

HOMŒOPATHIC TREATMENT OF ASTHMA

Remedy	Pathology	Time	Comments
Arsenicum	Acute Chronic	1-2 a.m.	Restless, fearful, < cold, > rocking, burning pains.
Kali carb	Acute	2-3 a.m.	Vomiting, < drinking, < motion, cutting pains. H/O Coryza which sets off the attacks
Natrum sulph	Acute Chronic	4-5 a.m.	< wet weather. Green discharge. Pain in lower left lobe
Ipecac	Acute		With nausea.
Oxygen 1M	Acute		Immediate first aid in 1m potency.
Cuprum met.	Acute		Spasm, cyanosis, violent attacks, clenched fingers and thumbs.
Agaricus	Chronic	< night.	The cough and spasm ends in a sneeze, coughs up little balls of snot.
Lycopodium	Chronic		
Medorrhinum	Chronic	< day. < night.	The 'usual' nosode. Choking cough, > lying on face, < lying down, > lying on stomach, feels cold and heat. << wet, damp, thunder, wants to be fanned.
Senega	Chronic		For asthma in the elderly, with rattling chest.
Apis	Acute	4-6 p.m.	< heat. Burning pains, oedema.
Rumex	Acute Chronic	Evening	< change in temperature, tickling cough, copious discharge.
See also			Tuberculinum, Ant tart., Lobelia, Veratrum viride.

Remember: Ventolin can be withdrawn at any time. Becotide is a steroid. Always advise your patients to consult their GP.

NB This table (as ever) is only a rough guide – a place to start looking; asthma is generally a deep-seated disease and may require deep, constitutional remedies.

FURTHER READING

P S Kamthan

Specific Remedies for Respiratory and Cardiac Diseases

B Jain Publishers

ISBN 81-8056-255-7

www.homeopathic.com

Gatchell

Diseases of the Lungs

B Jain Publishers

ISBN 81-8056-272-7

F Bernoville

Diseases of the Respiratory and Digestive System in Children

B Jain Publishers

ISBN 81-7021-389-4

Paul Herscu

The Homeopathic Treatment of Children

North Atlantic Books

ISBN 1-55643-090-6

P Sivaraman

Asthma Cured with Homœopathic Medicines

B Jain Publishers

ISBN 81-7021-356-8

NOTES

NOTES

CONTENTS

THE ENDOCRINE SYSTEM

The Endocrine System is composed of a number of organs and tissues of the body that collectively release substances known as hormones.

Definitions for this page
Hormones are chemical substances formed in the body that are carried in the bloodstream to affect another part of the body, like 'messenger' molecules that help coordinate the actions of various tissues. They are made in one part of the body and transported, via the bloodstream, to other parts, where they have a specific effect on certain cells. An example is thyroid hormone, produced by the thyroid gland in the neck, which affects growth, temperature regulation, metabolic rate, and other body functions.

Endocrine organs are also known as ductless glands because their secretions are released directly into the bloodstream. So this is in contrast to exocrine glands, which discharge their secretions on such external or internal surface tissues as those of the skin, the lining of the stomach, or of the lining of the pancreatic ducts.

The endocrine glands and their hormones regulate the growth, development, and function of certain tissues and co-ordinate many of the metabolic processes within the body. The endocrine system is the 'great forgotten system' for many practitioners, so it is well worth making the effort to understand its workings. Pathologies that affect hormone regulation can be far-reaching, hard to identify, and profound. An endocrine system that has been returned to normal regulation can 'solve' a huge number of apparently unrelated disorders.

Hormone-producing tissues may be classified into three groups:

- Purely endocrine glands, which function solely in hormone production.
- Endo-exocrine glands, that produce other types of secretions as well as hormones.
- Certain non-glandular tissues, such as the autonomic nerves, which produce hormone-like substances.

THE PITUITARY GLAND

The pituitary gland, or hypophysis, consists of three lobes, the anterior lobe, the intermediate lobe (which in primates is present for only a short part of the life span), and the posterior lobe. It is situated at the base of the brain and has been called the "master-controlling gland" of the body.

The anterior and the posterior lobes of the pituitary secrete different hormones.

The anterior lobe secretes various hormones that stimulate the function of other endocrine glands; amongst the stream of hormones flowing from the anterior lobe are the following:

- Adrenocorticotropic hormone, or ACTH, which stimulates the adrenal cortex. More specifically, it stimulates secretion of glucocorticoids such as cortisol. Very crudely the glucocorticoids assist the body to manage stress.
- Thyroid-stimulating hormone, or thyrotropin, known as TSH, which stimulates that gland to synthesize and release thyroid hormones. The general functions of the thyroid hormones are to increase oxidative metabolism and enhance growth and development and nervous system maturation in children.
- Follicle-stimulating hormone (FSH), which stimulates the maturation of ovarian follicles and is also critical for sperm production.
- Luteinising hormone (LH), which stimulate the sex glands.
- Prolactin, which, with other special hormones, influences milk production.

In addition, the anterior pituitary is the source of growth hormone, also called somatotropin, which promotes the development of body tissues, particularly of bone matrix and muscle, and influences carbohydrate metabolism.

Bone Matrix
Bones consist of living cells in a calcium carbonate matrix. It is the matrix that makes up the main bone material. In the event of a broken bone, the cells are brought out of semi-stasis to repair the matrix. The matrix comprises the major constituent of bone. It has both inorganic and organic parts. The inorganic is mainly crystalline mineral salts and calcium, which are present in the form of hydroxylapatite. The organic part of matrix is mainly Type 1 collagen.

The anterior pituitary also secretes a hormone called Melanocyte-stimulating hormone, which regulates the intensity of pigmentation in pigmented cells. In the 1970s, scientists found that the anterior pituitary also produces substances called endorphins. These are peptides that act on the peripheral and central nervous systems to reduce sensitivity to pain.

So we can see that even disturbances in this one area could potentially cover an enormous range of disorders – disorders that we often try to treat 'at face value'. Treatment will often be much more effective if the underlying disturbance is perceived and the underlying cause is addressed.

Pituitary functioning may be disturbed by such conditions as:

- Tumours
- Blood poisoning
- Blood clots
- Infectious diseases
- Under-secretion of the anterior lobe

Where the anterior lobe is not secreting sufficiently any of the following pathologies may emerge:

- Dwarfism
- Acromicria
- Simmonds's disease
- Fröhlich's syndrome

Definitions for this page
Dwarfism occurs when anterior pituitary deficiencies occur during childhood. Acromicria, in which the bones of the extremities are small and delicate, results when the deficiency occurs after puberty. Simmond's disease, which is caused by extensive damage to the anterior pituitary, is characterised by premature ageing, loss of hair and teeth, anaemia, and emaciation; it can be fatal. Both anterior pituitary deficiency and a lesion of the posterior lobe or hypothalamus cause Frölich's syndrome, also called adiposogenital dystrophy. The result is obesity, dwarfism and retarded sexual development.

Inevitably those glands that are under the influence of anterior pituitary hormones are also affected by any anterior pituitary deficiency.

GIANTISM AND ACROMEGALY

Gigantism results from the overproduction of growth hormone during childhood or adolescence. The arms and legs grow especially long, and height can surpass 2.4m (8 ft). The disorder is caused by a pituitary tumor that, if untreated, usually kills the patient by early adulthood.

If the tumor develops after growth of the long bones is complete, the result is a condition called acromegaly, characterized by a long face, jutting jaw, and large feet and hands.

CUSHING'S SYNDROME

This is a collection of symptoms that arise from an excess of corticosteroids in the blood stream (usually of iatrogenic cause, although there is a possibility of a tumour being the cause). Symptoms include discoloured skin (reddened), acne, bloating, fat shoulders, brittle bones and high BP.

Definitions for this page
An iatrogenic disease is one that has resulted from treatment - either as an unforeseen or an inevitable side effect.

UNDER-SECRETION OF THE POSTERIOR LOBE

Where the posterior lobe is not secreting sufficiently, diabetes insipidus may develop. Diabetes insipidus is caused by the inability of the kidneys to conserve water, which leads to frequent urination and pronounced thirst. This occurs because insufficient hormone ADH is being produced.

CONVENTIONAL TREATMENT FOR PITUITARY DISORDERS

Treatment may be directed towards replacing the hormones of the targeted gland or, where a tumour is suspected, to the tumour as well as to hormone replacement therapy. In the case of a tumour the options are usually surgery or radiation therapy.

HOMŒOPATHIC TREATMENT FOR PITUITARY DISORDERS

In treating any glandular disorder it is well worth remembering that Robin Murphy has included a whole chapter on Glands in his Repertory – starting on page 813, sadly he devotes no rubrics at all to the Pituitary Gland, so we have to look harder for remedies for specific conditions.

Dwarfism is contained in the repertory (under Constitutions, p. 311) and the remedies suggested include (black type) *Baryta carb, Calc phos, Medorrhinum, Silica* and *Sulphur*. Oddly there is only a small type mention for *Syphilinum*, which would perhaps be many people's first choice. Certainly it would be very important to look closely at the miasmatic picture.

Acromicria is not mentioned at all in Murphy, but again you would be looking to the miasmatic picture and to remedies that strengthen the bone structure (perhaps *Calc Phos* as a tissue salt, etc.)

Simmonds's disease: if this disease strikes before puberty the patient will remain Peter Pan-like.... short and sexually undeveloped; this should give plenty of scope for prescribing and again we would perhaps be looking at *Baryta carb* and *Calc carb*.

Fröhlich's syndrome is also going to give us scope to treat with the remedies above, and (as usual) any well-chosen constitutional remedy.

DIETARY TREATMENT FOR PITUITARY DISORDERS

The amino acid Arginine is necessary for the normal functioning of the Pituitary Gland. It is required for the synthesis and release of the Pituitary Gland's growth hormone. Arginine has a number of functions, these include:

- Aids immunisation response
- Help in wound healing
- Helps to metabolise stored body fat
- Tones up muscle tissue
- Increases sperm count

The best natural sources of Arginine are nuts, popcorn, carob, gelatin, chocolate, brown rice, oatmeal, raisins, sunflower and sesame seeds, whole wheat bread and all protein rich foods.

Interestingly Arginine-rich foods are contraindicated for anyone who has herpes.

HOMŒOPATHIC TREATMENT

As we've seen, the activity of the pituitary gland has an enormous impact on the body. Consequently there's any number of remedies that could be useful if this area is perceived as the focus of a disease. As usual it would be wise to take the case and tailor a remedy to the patient's needs. Sometimes a 'support remedy' can help as well. These two have been shown to help – you'll have to do your own research to choose between them:

- *Pituitrin 30*
- *Baryta carb 30*

THE HYPOTHALAMUS

The hypothalamus consists of a tiny cluster of nerve cells located at the centre of the base of the brain.

This organ serves as a link between the autonomic nervous system and the endocrine system.

The hypothalamus is responsible for many body functions. Its aim is to integrate and ensure appropriate response to stimuli. It regulates hunger, thirst, sleep, and wakefulness.

It also plays an important role in the regulation of most of the involuntary mechanisms of the body, including body temperature, sexual drive, and the female menstrual cycle. The hypothalamus also regulates the work of the pituitary gland. It secretes an antidiuretic hormone (one that controls the excretion of water) named vasopressin, which is stored in the posterior lobe of the pituitary gland. So vasopressin controls the amount of water secreted by the kidneys and raises blood pressure.

The posterior lobe of the pituitary also stores another hormone secreted by the hypothalamus. This hormone, known as oxytocin, stimulates muscular contractions, especially of the uterus – notably during childbirth, and ejection of milk from lactating mammary glands.

PATHOLOGY OF THE HYPOTHALAMUS

Disorders of the hypothalamus are usually reflected in the target glands or organs and therefore will be discussed in that order.

THE ADRENAL GLANDS

The adrenal glands (suprarenal glands) curve over the top of each kidney in the abdomen. Although it appears to be one organ, it is actually two small glands, each weighing about 1/4 ounce (7 grams). The adrenal medulla (inner part or zona glomerulosa) is an agent of the sympathetic nervous system and is activated by nerve impulses.

The adrenal cortex (the outer part, or zona fasciculata) is a true endocrine gland activated by adrenocorticotrophic hormone (ACTH) sent out from the pituitary gland.

THE ADRENAL MEDULLA

The adrenal medulla secretes hormones to help the body reduce stress (notably epinephrine and norepinepherine). When the sympathetic nervous system reacts to intense emotions, such as fright or anger, large amounts of the hormone are released. This has a number of effects, including:

- Stimulation of cardiac action
- Increasing blood pressure

It affects constriction and dilation of blood vessels

And also affects constriction of musculature

This may cause the "fight or flight" reaction, in which blood pressure rises, the pupils widen, and blood is shunted to the most vital organs and to the skeletal muscles. The heart is also stimulated. This valuable response is most often seen in these 'tamer' times when we are driving.

THE ADRENAL CORTEX

The adrenal cortex secretes two hormones: cortisol and aldosterone. These hormones are known collectively as corticosteroids. They help the body reduce stress and are essential for life. Cortisol is an energy generator. It regulates conversion of carbohydrates into glucose and directs reserves to the liver. It also suppresses inflammation. Aldosterone regulates the mineral and water balance of the body. It prevents excessive loss of water through the kidneys and maintains the balance between sodium and potassium in the blood stream. This balance is important to the ability of the muscles to contract.

The adrenal outer layer, or cortex, secretes about 30 steroid hormones, but only a few are secreted in significant amounts. It produces three types of kinds of corticosteroid hormones that affect carbohydrate metabolism (cortisol for example), electrolyte metabolism (such as aldosterone) and the sex glands (both oestrogens and androgens).

CUSHING'S SYNDROME

Technically speaking Cushing's syndrome can be described as a disorder of the adrenal glands (although more commonly it is seen as one related to the pituitary gland as previously discussed). It's a moot point – where one hormonal imbalance causes another one, where is the pathology located?

PHAECHROMOCYTOMA

The adrenal glands can also be subject to tumour, most common being Phaechromocytoma (Phaose = grey, chromos = colour, cytos = cell). This tumour is benign and attacks the central part of the gland, the medulla. Because the medulla is responsible for the production of adrenaline and noradrenalin, it is these hormones that are overproduced. Naturally enough this results in palpitations, perspiration, headache and hypertension. A permanent state of preparedness for fight or flight!

DIETARY AND LIFESTYLE TREATMENTS FOR ADRENAL DISORDERS

There are dietary considerations in the treatment of adrenal dysfunction – substances that further stress the adrenals should preferably be avoided; these include:

- Tea
- Coffee
- Cigarettes
- Chocolate

In dealing with these (and a million other stressors) the body has to make some sacrifices. Digestion is slowed down as is routine repair and maintenance work. Prolonged stress is associated with speeding up the ageing process. It is also associated with upsetting the thyroid balance (as we shall see later), which means that the metabolism slows down and there is weight gain. Calcium balance can also be affected – resulting in arthritis, and the balance of sex hormones can be disrupted – resulting in more rows with your partner which causes more stress which … and so on. The long-term effect of the over-stimulated system, almost any system, is that it will under-function.

All hormones need nutrients for their production and adrenaline needs vitamins B3 (niacin), B12 and C. Corticosol (which is a natural anti-inflammatory substance) needs B5. The higher the stress of the system, the more the need for these vitamins.

The inevitable corollary to all this is that the only way to properly maintain health is to (as much as possible) avoid stressful situations. It is the duty of a good practitioner to provide their patients with enough evidence to make informed decisions about their life. Sadly many of our patients will still persist in their stressful lives ("I've got no choice") and consequently much treatment will be damage limitation.

HOMŒOPATHY FOR TREATMENT OF ADRENAL DISORDERS

Ian Watson recommends, as Organ Support, the use of *Adrenal gland 6* or *Adrenalin 6*. Unsurprising choices really. If in doubt … take the case!

THE THYROID GLAND

The Thyroid Gland is the endocrine gland found in almost all vertebrate animals and so called because it is located in front of and on each side of the thyroid cartilage of the larynx. It secretes a hormone that controls metabolism and growth.

STRUCTURE AND SECRETIONS

The thyroid gland in human beings is a brownish-red organ having two lobes connected by an isthmus; it normally weighs about 28 g (about 1 oz.) and consists of cuboidal epithelial cells arranged to form small sacs known as vesicles or follicles.

The vesicles are supported by connective tissue that forms a framework for the entire gland. In the normal thyroid gland, the vesicles are usually filled with a colloid substance containing the protein thyroglobulin in combination with the two thyroid hormones thyroxine, also called tetraiodothyronine (T4), and triiodothyronine (T3).

The amount of thyroglobulin secreted by the thyroid is controlled by the thyroid-stimulating hormone (TSH) of the pituitary gland. Pituitary TSH, in turn, is regulated by a substance called thyroid-stimulating hormone releasing factor (TRF), which is secreted by the hypothalamus.

Thyroglobulin is especially rich in iodine. Although the thyroid gland constitutes about 0.5 percent of the total human body weight, it holds about 25 percent of the total iodine in the body, which is obtained from food and water in the diet. Iodine usually circulates in the blood as an inorganic iodide and is concentrated in the thyroid to as much as 500 times the iodide level of the blood.

PARATHYROID GLANDS

The parathyroids are found near or embedded in the thyroid gland. The parathyroid hormone regulates blood levels of calcium and phosphorus and stimulates bone reabsorption.

CANCER OF THE THYROID

Many different laboratory tests, including direct measurement of thyroxine and triiodothyronine, are used to test the activity of the thyroid gland. Thyroid scanning with radioiodine or technetium-99m is especially useful for detecting or ruling out cancer of the thyroid in persons who have a palpable nodule, or thyroid lump. In most cases thyroid cancers are slow growing and not fatal. The thyroid gland appears to be quite sensitive to irradiation: during the 1970s an increased incidence of thyroid cancer was found among people who had been treated early in life with X rays for such conditions as acne, ringworm, and tonsillitis.

THYROTOXICOSIS

Excessive production of thyroid hormones, called Hyperthyroidism, Thyrotoxicosis or Graves' disease, results in elevated metabolism and activity. Sometimes this condition is associated with abnormalities of the eye, including bulging eyes. Another term with which you may be familiar is Goitre.

Overactive thyroid is often a female complaint with an aetiology of shock, emotional trauma, etc. The symptoms as presented in practise may be as follows:

- increase in metabolic activity
- weight loss
- increase in appetite
- hot and sweaty sensation
- greasy and oily skin
- 'poor energy' or restless & unproductive energy
- nervousness, restlessness
- apprehension
- warm & sweaty handshake
- palpitations in the chest
- increased heart rate
- atrial fibrillation
- fine tremor of the hands
- bulging eyes
- change in menstrual cycle (irregular and less frequent)

Many of the above symptoms mimic those of anxiety and panic attacks – so Thyrotoxicosis may be misdiagnosed as an anxiety state.

CONVENTIONAL TREATMENT

Surgery is difficult in the case of the thyroid gland because of the surrounding nerves and carotid arteries, jugular vein etc. It is possible to remove part of the thyroid – partial thyroidectomy – and this can often be done. It is worth knowing that when a patient is told that part of the thyroid has been removed (sometimes called a sub-total thyroidectomy rather than partial) up to 90% may be removed. This is quite a large amount of thyroid to have to cope without. Surgery can lead to Thyroid Crisis where the gland goes into overdrive to try and compensate and huge amounts of thyroxine are released – this can be fatal.

Another conventional treatment is to administer an antithyroid drug, such as propylthiouracil, or a dose of radioactive iodine, which is concentrated in the thyroid gland and destroys some of the tissue.

HOMŒOPATHIC TREATMENT

Remedies to consider would be *Natrum mur, Iodum, Calc carb,* and *Fucus vesiculosus.*

Fucus Ves is one of the remedies that you would naturally think of to have an affinity for the thyroid gland (being as it is Sea Kelp and therefore stuffed with iodine) and potencies to consider would be:

- 4c which inhibits the organ
- 7c which regulates the organ
- 9c which stimulates the organ

MYXOEDEMA

This is an under-activity of the thyroid gland (hypothyroidism), and is characterised by lethargy and lowering of metabolism. It is generally slow and insidious in onset; thus it may go unnoticed for years. Patients display a range of symptoms as follows:

- slowness
- apathy
- lowered libido
- mental and physical dullness
- monotonous voice
- monosyllabic response
- poor appetite
- increased weight
- coarse, dry skin
- thin, brittle hair…which then falls out
- non-pitting oedema
- lowered blood pressure
- constipation
- hair growth on face

Hypothyroidism is subnormal activity of the thyroid gland. The condition called cretinism, which is more properly known as congenital hypothyroidism, is an inherited deficiency of thyroid function that occurs in about one in every 6000 births. In most instances, but not all, these infants grow up to be mentally retarded. Since early treatment can prevent retardation, Canadian researchers developed a test to detect the condition in newborns. In children the most obvious signs to look out for are: tongue sticking out, and a failure to thrive.

Allopathic treatment tends to be the use of thyroxine but this can lead to problems such as Ischaemic Heart Disease (and then myocardial infarction).

Remedies to consider include *Spongia, Calc carb, Baryta carb* and (again) *Fucus ves.*

DIETARY REGULATION OF THE THYROID

Thyroxine is made from tyrosine; the enzyme that converts one into the other is dependent on iodine and selenium, both of which can be taken as supplements (the former in Kelp or seaweed). The thyroid gland also produces a hormone that is responsible for maintaining calcium balance in the body. Calcitonin from the thyroid works in balance with parathhormone (PTH) from the parathyroid glands. PTH converts vitamin D into an active hormone that helps to increase available calcium. Most of the body's calcium is in the bones, but a small amount is in the blood – PTH stimulates the bones to give up calcium and Calcitonin puts calcium back into the bones. So vitamin D is a vital ingredient in this process. Don't forget that calcium is used in every single nerve and muscle reaction.

OTHER ENDOCRINE COMPONENTS

THE PINEAL GLAND

Also known as the Pineal Body, this is a small, cone-shaped projection from the top of the midbrain of most vertebrates, arising embryologically as an outgrowth of the brain.

The structure develops until the seventh year, when it is slightly larger than a pea; thereafter, throughout life, small mineral particles, particularly calcium, may be deposited in the pineal body. The mineral deposits can sometimes be seen in skull X-ray photographs.

Named after a French psychologist, Philippe Pinel, who first described the gland in the human brain, its functions are only slowly beginning to be understood. It has both neural and endocrine properties, and also light receptive properties. People who are completely unsighted and have no neural connection between the eyes and the brain are still able to detect some light;

it is thought therefore that the pineal gland has a function in this area. In mammals the pineal body is not thought to be light sensitive of itself, but a neural connection remains between the eyes and the gland. Thus the functions of the pineal body in an animal are linked with surrounding light levels.

The isolation of the hormone melatonin in 1958 has led to a further understanding of the pineal body. Animal studies show that the gland synthesises and secretes melatonin almost entirely at night, and that it ceases this function during the day. Melatonin, in turn, affects the functions of other endocrine organs such as the thyroid, adrenals, and gonads. Further experiments demonstrated that changes in the level of melatonin in the bodies of seasonally breeding animals affect their reproductive cycle, and further that decreases in melatonin brought about by artificial lighting can prolong breeding activity. The role of the pineal body in the control of these biorhythms is only beginning to be elaborated, but the suggestion remains that even non-seasonal breeders such as human beings are affected by its daily functions. The onset of puberty may, in fact, be triggered by changes in melatonin level.

ENDOCRINE CYCLES

The endocrine system exerts a regulatory action on the reproductive cycles, including the development of the gonads, their period of functional maturity, and their subsequent senescence, as well as the menstrual cycle and the gestation period.

Puberty, the time of sexual maturation, is marked by an increase in the secretion of pituitary gonad-stimulating hormones or gonadotropins, which cause maturation of the testes or ovaries and increased secretion of sex hormones. The sex hormones, in turn, affect the accessory sex organs and general development.

Puberty in the female is associated with the onset of menstruation and ovulation. Ovulation, the release of an ovum from an ovarian follicle, occurs approximately every 28 days at about the 10th to 14th day of the menstrual cycle in human beings. The first part of the cycle is marked by the actual menstrual period, averaging about three to five days, and by the maturation of the ovarian follicle under the influence of the follicle-stimulating hormone of the pituitary. After ovulation, the vacated follicle, under the influence of another pituitary hormone, forms an endocrine body known as the corpus luteum that secretes progesterone, oestrogen, and, probably during pregnancy, relaxin. Progesterone prepares the uterine lining for pregnancy; if it does not occur, the corpus luteum regresses, and the uterine lining, deprived of hormonal support, breaks down, resulting in menstrual bleeding. The rhythmic pattern of menstruation is explained by the reciprocal inhibitory-stimulative relationship between the oestrogens and the pituitary gonad-stimulating hormones.

If pregnancy occurs, the placental secretion of gonadotropins, progesterones, and oestrogens maintains the corpus luteum and the uterine lining and prepares the mammary glands for milk production, or lactation. Secretion of oestrogens and progesterone is high during pregnancy, reaching a peak just before childbirth. Lactation begins shortly after the delivery, presumably as a result of changes in hormone balance following separation of the placenta.

With the progressive process of aging of the ovaries and decrease in ovarian oestrogen production, menopause occurs. Secretion of gonadotropins increases at this time, apparently as a result of lack of oestrogen inhibition. In the male the corresponding period is marked by a gradual reduction in androgen secretion.

OVARIES

The ovaries are the female gonads, which are paired, almond-shaped bodies situated on either side of the uterus. The ovarian follicles produce the ova, or eggs, and also secrete a group of hormones called oestrogens, which are necessary for the development of the reproductive organs and of such secondary sex characteristics as the distribution of fat, widening of the pelvis, mammary growth, and pubic and axillary hair.

Progesterone is another hormone produced by the ovaries, which has as its principal function the maintenance of pregnancy. It accomplishes this primarily by its effects on the lining of the uterus. Progesterone also acts in conjunction with oestrogens in promoting the growth and elasticity of the female genital tract. The ovaries elaborate a hormone called Relaxin, which acts to relax the cervix during childbirth, thus making delivery easier (allegedly).

TESTES

The male gonads, the testes, are paired, ellipsoid bodies suspended in the scrotum. The Leydig cells of the testes produce one or more male hormones called the androgens. The androgens, the most important of which is testosterone, stimulate the development of secondary sex characteristics, influence the growth of the prostate and seminal vesicles, and promote secretory activity of these structures. The testes also contain cells that produce sperm.

PANCREAS

The bulk of the pancreas consists of exocrine tissue that releases digestive juices into the duodenum. Distributed throughout this tissue are clusters of endocrine cells called the islets of Langerhans, which secrete insulin and another hormone known as glucagon.

Insulin affects carbohydrate, protein, and fat metabolism, increasing the rate of sugar utilisation and promoting formation of protein and storage of fat.

Glucagon temporarily raises blood-sugar levels, apparently by releasing glucose from the liver.

PLACENTA

The placenta, an organ formed during pregnancy from the membrane surrounding the foetus and the uterine lining, assumes certain endocrine functions of the pituitary gland and the ovaries that are important in the maintenance of pregnancy. It secretes the hormone called chorionic gonadotropin, a substance found in the urine during pregnancy and constituting the basis for pregnancy tests. The placenta produces the sex hormones progesterone and the oestrogens, a protein hormone with some of the characteristics of growth hormone, and lactogenic hormones (placental lactogen).

OTHER HORMONE SOURCES

Hormones and hormone-like substances are also produced by certain other body tissues. For example the kidneys secrete an agent called Renin, which activates the hormone angiotensin produced in the liver; this hormone in turn raises blood pressure, probably in part by stimulating the release of aldosterone by the adrenal glands. The kidneys also elaborate a hormone called erythropoietin, which stimulates the bone marrow to produce red blood cells. Regulatory hormones can be found in other systems too (especially the digestive system) in, frankly, too complex a way to be of practical use to us in this context.

TONSILLITIS

One area of related pathology worth having a look at tonsillitis; it is often forgotten that the tonsils are two bodies of lymphatic tissue which (loosely) constitute part of the overall glandular system.

It's important to have some 'tools' to deal with tonsillitis because of the frequency with which we see this complaint in clinic. Although a relatively common disease, tonsillitis is potentially quite damaging to the system, so (as ever) rapid and accurate prescribing would be a great plan.

Tonsillitis is an inflammation of the tonsils (and/or surrounding area) due to bacterial or viral infection.

CONVENTIONAL TREATMENT

This is customarily antibiotics or surgery, neither option being particularly desirable from a homœopathic perspective. It is commonly accepted that the tonsils form part of the body's immune system and that they can be a 'first line of defence'. So trying to help the patient to keep them would be highly favourable from a conventional and homœopathic viewpoint.

Although conventional treatment may seem a little aggressive, it is worth remembering that there is a range of potential sequelae (a disorder that results from a previous disease – 'that which follows on') to tonsillitis. In this case sequelae can include rheumatic fever (fever, arthritis going from joint to joint, and inflammation of the membrane surrounding the heart). Rheumatic fever can become chronic, and very debilitating; however it is very unlikely to occur if the patient is taking antibiotics. Frankly, there are times when one should consider the lesser of the evils, regardless of personal feelings. Another possible sequel to tonsillitis can be nephritis (sometimes called Bright's disease, especially in older literature) – an inflammation of the kidneys. Once again this can be a nasty complication, so be sure that your homœopathy is top notch.

HOMŒOPATHIC TREATMENT

Here are a few possibilities that may prove useful in treating tonsillitis – even when dealing with an acute disease there can never be a definitive list, but these have been shown to be helpful.

ALUMEN

Not to be confused with *Alumina*, this remedy is Potash Alum; Potassic Aluminic Sulphate. It is a remedy that is generally helpful for hardening and/or inflammation of glands (any glands), and is often characterised by a sensation of dryness and constriction. This is one of the 'sudden' remedies – there's usually a quickness of onset. For example the child goes to bed as normal, but during the night gets very ill, very quickly.

Obviously with this condition the tonsils would be inflamed, the uvula may appear elongated, and the oesophagus can go into spasm. This will make swallowing difficult, even swallowing liquids – highly inconvenient when you are dry and have a "constant desire to drink". This is a remedy that can spit up blood in the mornings, and there may be aetiology of a cold…maybe moving to a chest infection, and then to the tonsils.

BARYTA CARB

This is commonly thought of as an infancy or old age remedy, consequently these are the times of life it is most likely to be indicated. One of the things to look out for if you suspect that this may be the most appropriate remedy is that the mother may be unaware of the child's tonsillitis. This is because the child may always have swollen tonsils – it is, after all, one of the keynote symptoms of the remedy. These children are prone to quinsy (the exactly accurate name for which is 'peritonsillar abscess'), which we see quite commonly described in older homœopathic literature. Often the term quinsy seems to be interchangeable for tonsillitis, in fact though quinsy is a *complication* of tonsillitis in which the soft palette around the tonsils is swollen and pus filled.

Inevitably this makes swallowing pretty difficult – the conventional treatment may be surgical incision.

The relevant physical particulars of this remedy are that there is often a history of colds, many episodes of tonsillitis and/or quinsy, the throat is very sore and a strange sensation as if there were a plug in the throat (or I have heard it described "as if there were some food lodged there".)

BELLADONNA

This may well be the number one remedy for children with acute tonsillitis, and I need hardly reiterate the outstanding characteristics of this brilliant remedy (but here they are anyway) – intense heat, burning sensation, throbbing, and of course redness. In children there will be no thirst and (oddly) no anxiety, and the throat will look red and 'angry'. It will be difficult to swallow because of a strong sense of constriction, but there is a constant urge to swallow – they feel that they'll suffocate if they don't.

GUAIACUM OFFICINALE

This is a relatively small remedy, but it's well indicated for acute tonsillitis characterised by a burning in the throat, which is much worse for heat. It is said that *Guaiacum* has some of the qualities of *Apis, Baryta carb,* and *Belladonna* in that it has the redness of *Belladonna*, the oedema of *Apis*, and the inflammation, ulceration and suppuration of *Baryta carb*. So it would be a 'natural' to be amongst the possible choices for tonsillitis.

In tonsillitis, the right side is more likely to be the most affected, with swelling, a dark redness and aching or stitching pains. This is one of the remedies that has aching in the teeth, which may well be a concomitant to the tonsillitis.

HEPAR SULPH

Another candidate for the first choice for tonsillitis; the patient will be irritable, sensitive, and of course there is a tendency to suppuration. The outstanding sensation (in the throat) is likely to be that of a splinter, and patients will often complain that it hurts when they swallow and that the pain "goes right up into my ear". It is actually difficult for them to speak and/or swallow – sometimes they can't even swallow their own saliva.

LAC CANINUM

This is the remedy for the child who wakes up different from the previous night; they wake with a sore throat and the tonsils (especially the right one) are covered with ulcers and patches – these then spread to cover the left side. Next day the child is worse (unless they've had the brilliantly well-chosen remedy, of course) with a fever and chills, pains in the head, back, and limbs, and they're very, very restless. On observation you'll see that there is swelling in the neck glands and, naturally enough, the mother is anxious about this being meningitis.

This remedy also has the sensation of a lump in the throat but with *Lac caninum* the lump goes down when they swallow and then returns. The throat may also feel 'stiff'.

LACHESIS

This is another well-known remedy, whose main sphere of affinity can often be the throat. So it'd be a clear candidate for tonsillitis, the four relevant keynotes are:

- Worse during or after sleep
- Very sensitive to touch
- Left sided complaints (or those that go from left to right)
- Better for discharges

As the throat area is one of the affinities of the remedy, sore throats of every description may be helped by it. They can't bear any pressure round the neck and have difficulty swallowing. Strangely 'empty' swallowing is the most painful, swallowing liquids is not so bad, and swallowing solids is the least painful of all – kind of the reverse to what we'd expect. Unfortunately they may have an unquenchable thirst!

MERCURY

With this remedy the throat may feel dry and yet the mouth is full of saliva, so full that they can't speak clearly. There can be an accumulation of thick mucus in the throat, with a constant desire to swallow, which only aggravates. The throat is describes as sore, raw, smarting, and burning…with a strange sensation as if hot vapour were ascending from the stomach.

SILICA

Many homœopaths initial thoughts go to this remedy when tonsillitis is mentioned, and with good reason. Indeed Silica 12x is said by many to be a specific for severe tonsillitis. The symptoms include pains in the throat 'as if from the pricking of a pin', and swelling of the uvula and of the whole palette. It can be difficult to swallow – as if the whole throat were paralysed; so difficult indeed that food can come out of the nose.

Patients who need this remedy will probably have had previous episodes of quinsy (and/or tonsillitis) and all colds will tend to 'settle' in the throat, with concomitant swelling of the glands.

FURTHER READING

Adolf Voegeli MD

Homœopathic Prescribing

Thorsons Publishers Ltd.

ISBN 0-7225-03431

John Henry Clarke MD

A Clinical Repertory to the Dictionary of Materia Medica

B Jain Publishers

ISBN 81-7021-066-6

Didier Grandgeorge MD

Homeopathic Remedies for the Stages of Life

North Atlantic Books

ISBN 1-55643-409-X

Martin Miles

Homœopathy and Human Evolution

Winter Press

ISBN 1-874581-00-2

Dua Shiv

Know and Solve Thyroid Problems

B Jain Press

ISBN 81-8056-471-1

NOTES

NOTES

CONTENTS

THE MALE REPRODUCTIVE SYSTEM

The male reproductive system is responsible for generating, storing, and transporting the genetic material contained in the sperm cells, or spermatozoa.

The chief organs include the testicles (or testes), the epididymides, the vas deferens, the ejaculatory duct, the urethra, and the penis. Auxiliary organs include the bulbo-urethral (Cowper's) glands, the prostate gland, and the seminal vesicles.

Spermatozoa (sperm cells) contain the chromosomes that will combine with those of the ovum, or egg (produced by the female reproductive system), to form the embryo of a new human.

ACCESSORY GLANDS

Among the glands accessory to the reproductive process are those that provide a fluid medium in which the spermatozoa may live, those that produce mucus which reduces friction during copulation, and those that emit apparently alluring odours to members of the opposite sex.

The seminal vesicles of the male have already been mentioned as organs that secrete mucus. The most important male accessory gland is the prostate gland, a compound gland about the size of a chestnut located at the base of the urethra where the urethra leaves the bladder and enters the penis. The prostate secretes a thin milky fluid with a characteristic odour; this fluid constitutes the greater part of the semen that is deposited in the female vagina and that contains the spermatozoa.

PATHOLOGY

Although we'll be looking at specific conditions and their treatment, both conventionally and homœopathically, there will often (always?) be a strong psychological component to these cases that should be taken into account. Many men see their genitalia as defining them as a man. Diseases and dysfunction of the penis therefore can have an enormous impact on the psyche. (Of course this is also true of a woman's relationship with her primary and secondary sex characteristics), so… on to the pathology:

BALANITIS

This can also be known as Balanoposthitis and is a generalised infection of the glans penis and foreskin. It is commonly caused by bacterial and yeast infections under the foreskin (naturally if your patient is circumcised there has been a misdiagnosis).

Complications can include:

MEATAL STRICTURE

The meatus is the opening of the urethra; and stricture is a narrowing of any tubular structure – the symptom you're looking for here is pain or difficulty in passing urine.

PHIMOSIS

This is a narrowing of the opening of the foreskin and is a particular problem because if the foreskin cannot be drawn back, there is a greater tendency to infection – and this results in further narrowing. In extremis the conventional treatment is circumcision, for which the number one remedy is *Staphysagria.*

PARAPHIMOSIS

This is condition where the foreskin can be pulled back over the glans penis, but then gets stuck there. Allegedly a very painful experience, which is remedied conventionally by 'manual replacement' under local or even general anaesthetic. Again the eventual treatment may be circumcision, without which the patient may expect a recurrence.

CANCER

Another complication that can also be a follow on from Balanitis

CONVENTIONAL TREATMENT

The treatment of Balanitis (if it is not too severe) is centered on an improvement in hygiene. A guarantee that your children won't suffer can be gained by either having a girl, or by early circumcision. The latter will also improve the boy's partner's chances of avoiding various cancers.

HOMŒOPATHIC TREATMENT OF INFLAMMATION

Homœopathic treatment needs to be swift and effective so it's important to be quite specific about exactly where the inflammation is. There are plenty of remedies available to treat inflammation of the penis (see page 1241 onward in Murphy's Repertory), but he is very specific as to the precise area that is inflamed. As close inspection may be awkward for both practitioner and patient, careful questioning is vital.

Here is a table showing some of the top remedies for inflammation of the penis. Remember – you'll need to be sure about some of the 'deeper' symptoms as well as the simple characteristics of the inflammation; consequently some of this is included here.

Remedy	Characteristics	Comment
Apis	Stinging darting pains. Red rosy hue. Oedema. Constricted sensation.	Apis is a remedy, which has increased sexual desire. Check whether this precedeed the infection. Also check for swelling and oedema of the testes.
Arsenicum	Restlessness. < night. Burning pains. Fearful, frightful, worried.	The glans can be swollen, cracked and described as 'bluish'. Also the patient is afraid of something worse than mere inflammation.
Cantharis	Violent inflammation of the sexual organs. Intolerable constant urging to urinate. < coffee.	The patient has greatly increased sexual desire (before or despite inflammation.) Frequent painful erections. Premature ejaculation too. They can be worse for sex.
Cinnabaris (red sulphide of mercury)	Swollen penis – can imitate gonorrhoea apparently. Redness, swelling and violent itching. Foetid and corrosive sweats between the thighs and scrotum when walking.	These are patients with a strong sexual desire. All their desires are exaggerated – sex, food and drink. Strong erections in the evening.
Rhus tox	Tearing pains. Great restlessness. Profuse eruptions on the penis, so that the urethra closes from the swelling.	These patients have their strongest desire in the morning, although they get erections at night. It is often accompanied by a desire to urinate.
Sulphur	Itching genitals – on going to bed, Inflammation with burning Cracks and redness. Weakness of genital function with icy blueness.	They have got an infection because hygiene is poor. Impotence and/or premature ejaculation all of which is very embarrassing to them.

PRIAPISM

Priapism is "a painful, persistent and abnormal erection unaccompanied by sexual desire or excitation" (Mercke Manual, 17th Edition). It seems that our conventional friends poorly understand the mechanisms of Priapism, but there is general agreement that they probably involve both vascular and neurological abnormalities. In some instances priapism can be secondary to prolonged sexual activity.

It has also been associated with quite a long list of other disorders; including leukaemia, sickle cell anaemia, pelvic haematoma (blood clots), cerebrospinal disease (e.g. syphilis or tumour), genital infection and inflammation (including cystitis). Priapism can also be an unwanted side effect of some drugs – including antihypertensives, chlorpromazine, anticoagulants, and corticosteroids. The reason for this huge list of associations is that the literature says that Priapism is relatively common. Yet you hear very little of it. This is a common dichotomy in men's health, there is very little available literature – notably in homœopathy – and yet many of the complaints are not rare.

Prognosis and Conventional Treatment

Prognosis for recovery of sexual functioning is poor unless treatment is prompt and effective. Some cases respond to vasoactive drugs administered directly. Neurogenic priapism may be alleviated by continuous spinal anaesthesia; otherwise the situation may be remedied by 'decompression', this means using large-bore needles and even then erection usually recurs.

In general there is a hope that something underlies the condition that can be readily identified and **that** condition can be treated.

HOMŒOPATHIC TREATMENT

We need, once again, to be quite specific about treating problems with erections. For the best possible outcome, it isn't good enough to give a remedy and wait a few weeks; we need to be acting quickly and be prepared to change remedies regularly if no appreciable difference is noted. I suggest you have a look in Murphy's Repertory. There are (how can I put this) a large number of erections, from page 1233 onward.

We would need to consider rubrics such as 'Erections continued' but there are others there which may be worth pondering on, (not just for priapism) including:

- Erections, troublesome
- Erections, too easy
- Erections, after eating
- Erections, excessive
- Erections, fruitless
- Erections, intolerable
- Erections, lying back on

- Erections, painful
- Erections, during pollutions
- Erections, seldom
- Erections, during supper
- Erections, with toothache
- Erections, while urinating
- Erections, while walking

The two major remedies to consider for priapism are *Hydrophobinum* and *Cantharis*. Hydrophobinum (*Lyssin* – the nosode of rabies) is lascivious and has strong erections without sexual excitement or thoughts and is apparently useful for priapism in stallions.

Cantharis can have painful swelling of the penis and/or painful swelling of the testes. This is also one of the remedies with increased desire but has pain after coition – burning pain in the urethra.

DISORDERS OF THE SCROTUM

Again, in general, this isn't something you hear a lot about, but there are a wide and bewildering array of things that can go wrong with this organ – here are just a few:

SCROTAL ABSCESSES

Nasty and painful – these can drain spontaneously, but conventionally most require surgery. Surgery is usually an orchidectomy (removal of the testes) so if you can do something homœopathically it will often appeal to the patient more than this rather radical solution. The remedies to consider are the usual suspects; *Hepar sulph, Mercury, Silica*, but also *Stillingia sylvatica* (whose common name – rather alarmingly – is Queen's Delight). This latter remedy has been used for syphilis and it has an affinity for the genito-urinary organs.

HYDROCELE

Hydrocele is a common intrinsic scrotal mass that results from excessive accumulation of sterile fluid. This accumulation can be due to overproduction or poor reabsorption. It usually appears as a painless scrotal swelling which can be transilluminated (this means that it is visible by shining a bright light through the sac – for people who really should get out more). Some men can get a little pain from the mass, but there are no signs of inflammation in most cases. Any man who has a Hydrocele will be worried sick prior to diagnosis – so be alert. Treatment of persistent Hydrocele (with symptoms – there's no point in treating it if asymptomatic) is by surgery.

Homœopathically there are a number of remedies – see Murphy page 1240 – and the main suspects are *Apis, Clematis, Graphites, Iodum, Pulsatilla, Rhododendron,* and *Silica.* More importantly than treatment though is getting the patient off to the doctors to get a diagnosis.

INGUINAL HERNIA

This can extend into the scrotal compartment and will be another cause for concern for your patient. A notable feature of inguinal herniation is that the mass will often be reduced when the patient lies down. Surgery is the usual conventional treatment because, if left alone, complications (such as strangulation) can occur.

Although this condition can have its signs and symptoms in the scrotal compartment we look it up under abdomen, hernia, inguinal (p. 27 in Murphy). The two big remedies are *Lycopodium* and *Nux vomica*...often thought of as major 'male' remedies. If the hernia becomes strangulated (while on the way to the doctors) your patient may benefit from *Belladonna, Opium* or a bit more *Nux vom.*

VARIOCELE

This is a collection of large veins – usually in the left scrotum and the sensation (if you can tease this information from your patient) is that if feels like "a bag of worms". For diagnostic purposes it should be present in the standing position, but absent when lying down. It can be associated with infertility, so the condition should be considered of major importance, especially for younger men. Conventional treatment, once again, is by surgery.

Homœopathically you'll be considering the 'chap's remedies' again; *Nux vom* and *Lycopodium* as well as *Sulphur*. Other choices include *Collinsonia canadensis* (Stone root), which has variocele with extreme constipation – in fact it has male sexual problems with constipation and piles. If the variocele is the result of a strain, then (as ever) the first choice remedy is *Ruta.*

GENITAL TRAUMA

It can happen that injuries of the penis or scrotum are penetrating or perforating but it is much more likely that they will be crushing blows and avulsion (avulsion means tearing or forcible separation of a part of a structure).

Testicular trauma, for example is usually secondary to physical combat of some kind. Avulsion injuries are more common among industrial and farm workers where clothing gets caught in machinery. The other cause of avulsion is excessive trauma during sex.

Conventionally (for those of you interested) avulsed skin should be cooled and reapplied as quickly as possible – even a completely transected penis can be reattached successfully – as John Bobbit can testify. If the testicles/whole scrotum are avulsed then treatment involves burying the testicles if possible, under the skin of the upper thighs or lower abdomen (the hope being that hormonal function can be retained).

Homœopathic remedies should be the ones that you usually think of for trauma – *Arnica, Bellis, Hypericum, Ruta*, and so forth.

ERECTILE DYSFUNCTION

This is the more diplomatic way of naming impotence. I'll dwell on this area for a little while because you 'should' see it commonly in practice. 52% of men age between 40 and 70 experience impotence. So over half of your male patients in this age range, statistically, will suffer. Ask yourself this: 'how many of them will tell you?' And if the answer is 'not many', then how can you find out if it's a problem?

AETIOLOGY

As usual it is very important that we seek an aetiology – this is especially true in erectile dysfunction. Because the symptoms are common, it's the cause that needs to be individualised. It is fairly rare that impotency is **primary** (ie. the man has never been able to attain or sustain an erection). Primary impotency is generally a psychological problem – related to sexual guilt, fear of intimacy, depression, severe anxiety states and so forth. Sometimes primary dysfunction is biogenic – usually associated with low testosterone levels.

Secondary impotency occurs when a man who could previously perform no longer can. More than 90% of these cases are organic to some degree. The major cause of dysfunction is vascular, other causes are hormonal, drug use (often non-prescribed, don't forget), and neurological. Any transient dysfunction can lead to a psychological component and this is then added to the case and to the cause. One thing to bear in mind is that dysfunction can be situational, involving place, time, a particular partner, or damage to self-esteem. Merck's Manual puts the conventional approach well – "The psychological factors that may accompany organic disorders cannot be overlooked and must be considered in every case. They may be the cause or the consequences of erectile dysfunction". Absolutely.

VASCULAR CAUSES

The major vascular problems include atherosclerotic diseases of the penile arteries – important for us to know, because we need to treat the cardiovascular system. (Atherosclerosis, remember, is a disease of the arteries wherein fatty plaques develop on the inner walls and thus block the flow of blood).

The venous system can also be a problem with inadequate impedance of the venous flow (venous leaks).

Conditions which affect the arterial and venous flow can accelerate dysfunction – the main two being diabetes and smoking.

Smoking increases the risk of erectile dysfunction by around 50% for men in their 30s and 40s. Smoking is a major and avoidable hazard for sexual health.

Given that two of the three main side effects of smoking on erectile function are acute responses to nicotine, immediate improvements on stopping smoking are possible. Cigarettes sold in Thailand now carry impotence warnings, and the idea is also under consideration in Hong Kong.

The damage caused by smoking to male sexual health also includes:

- Reduced volume of ejaculate
- Lowered sperm count
- Abnormal sperm shape
- Impaired sperm motility

HORMONAL AND NEUROLOGICAL COMPONENTS

Hormonal problems can cause dysfunction and if you think this may be causal, then the patient should be shipped off to the doctors for a testosterone check. Also several neurological disorders may have erectile dysfunction as part of the picture – these include MS, Stroke, Epilepsy, and spinal cord injuries. It is also worth noting that 40% of men having prostate operations experience difficulty with maintaining an erection after treatment.

DRUGS

Many of the drugs that are commonly used may impede erections. Some of these are shown in the table here:

Class	Drugs
Antihypertensives	Beta blockers
Central acting drugs	Any acting on the central nervous system.
Diuretics	Frusemide
False Neurotransmitters	Methyldopa
Psychotropics	MAOI's (Monoamine oxidase inhibitors), other antidepressants
CNS depressants	Sedatives, alcohol, opiates, cocaine, narcotics
Miscellaneous	Anti-cancer drugs, cimetidine

CONVENTIONAL TREATMENT

The underlying cause is as vital for the conventional practitioner as it is for homœopaths. Treatments include mechanical devices, surgery (implants), injections of various types, a medical vacuum device, and various oral drugs – including the famous Viagra.

HOMŒOPATHIC TREATMENT

Once again – you must get to the root cause. So as a guideline here are a few suggestions gathered by causation:

INJURY

Where there's a history of injury or blow to affected part, go with the usual number one trauma remedy, *Arnica*. Clarke says that it is useful in low potency (3c) given quite frequently – he says 4 hourly. By this I take it to mean that he is talking about a recent trauma. If the pathogeneses is more distant I would recommend higher potency, perhaps less frequently.

SPINAL INJURY

If the cause is spinal injury give *Hypericum* 1x 4 hourly and apply a liniment consisting of equal parts *Hypericum* tincture, spirit of wine, and distilled water to the affected part of the spine.

SIMPLE IMPOTENCE

Agnus castus 3x at 4 hourly intervals.

Impotence with wasting of the testicles

Kali brom 3x.

DUE TO SEXUAL EXCESS

Phosphoric acid.

AS PART OF A SYNDROME

When the patient is irritable, depressed, has constipation and/or other digestive disorders; *Nux vomica* 3x, 4 hourly.

LONG-TERM IMPOTENCE

Lycopodium 30 at 8 hourly intervals. In my experience this is the number one remedy for long-term impotence, and you may well find that you know nothing about the problem until you've given the remedy and the patient comes back with their presenting complaint (digestive disorders etc.) cured, and then they tell you that their libido is back too.

IF ALL ELSE FAILS

Clarke recommends *Selenium* 6c, 4 hourly and/or *Bufo* 30 – 200 night and morning.

Of course Robin Murphy has a whole lot of suggestions, see page 1240. His black type additions to the above list are *Baryta carbonica, Caladium*, a couple of *Calcs – Calc carb and Calc sulph, China, Conium, Medorrhinum, Phosphorus, Selenium, Sepia* (interestingly), and *Sulphur* (of course).

He only has one remedy for chronic impotency – *Lycopodium*, also the only remedy for older men. And it is worth studying the smaller rubrics – they can be a great help in this situation. There are a few remedies that have been helpful for diabetics, several for suppressed gonorrhoea (take the case well), and from abuse of tobacco – again *Lycopodium*, but also *Caladium*. In theory if you treat this condition well, you should have a huge number of men beating a path to your clinic.

FURTHER READING

George Vithoulkas **A New Model of Health and Disease**
North Atlantic Books
ISBN 1-55643-087-6 **www.homeopathyhome.com**

M L Tyler **Pointers to the Common Remedies**
B Jain Publishers
ISBN 81-7021-036-4

Ahmed Sayeed **Male Sexual Disorders**
B Jain Publishers
ISBN :81-7021-836-5

Tom Mettyear **Understanding Men's Vitatlity - Natural Solutions that Really Work**
Neal's Yard Press (an imprint of Winter Press)
ISBN 9781905830060

J P H Berjeau **The Homœopathic Treatment of Syphilis, Gonorrhoea, and Urinary Diseases**
B Jain Publishers
ISBN 81-7021-650-8

NOTES

NOTES

CONTENTS

THE FEMALE REPRODUCTIVE SYSTEM

The female reproductive system is responsible for generating the ovum, or egg, for storing the fertilized ovum, and nourishing the gestating embryo and foetus.

The chief organs include the ovaries, the uterus, vagina, and the Fallopian tubes. External (vulvar) organs include the labia majora, the labia minora, the mons pubis, the clitoris, the vestibule, and the greater vestibular cleft.

The ovum, or egg, contains the female's contribution to the genetic make-up of the new child (in other words the good bits, the looks, the brains, the sensitivity and so on), and is generated in the ovaries. The newly-generated ovum is passed through the fimbriated extremity of a Fallopian tube, into the Fallopian tube and there is fertilized by a spermatozoon (sperm cell).

During sexual arousal, a fluid created by the male's seminal vesicles and the prostate gland combines with the sperm cells to create semen, which is carried through the urethra and out of the opening, or meatus, in the end of the erect penis. When the semen is deposited in the female vagina, the spermatozoa swim through the uterus to the Fallopian tube, where it fertilizes the ovum, or egg. The fertilized egg travels down the Fallopian tube within the next three days and becomes attached to the wall of the uterus (womb). There, during pregnancy, the fertilized egg will be nourished and will develop into the embryo and, later, the foetus. Once fully developed (after about 40 weeks), muscular contractions (labour) will push the foetus out of the womb.

MENSTRUAL CYCLE

The menstrual cycle is the change that the female reproductive organs undergo about every 28 days beginning at puberty, usually between ages 11 and 14. It is the process in which an egg ripens in the ovaries and is released for fertilization. At the same time, a change occurs in the lining of the uterus, the endometrium, to prepare it for implantation of the fertilized egg. If fertilization does not take place, the endometrium breaks down, producing the menstrual flow, or period, and the cycle begins again. Different stages of the process are triggered by hormones (chemical messengers), two of which are secreted by the pituitary gland and two by the ovaries.

THE MENSTRUAL CYCLE – SIMPLE HORMONAL OVERVIEW

Conventionally the first day of the menstrual cycle is defined as the first day of bleeding. At this point all hormonal levels are pretty low and steady. The second stage is called the follicular phase or the proliferative phase. This is the time that the egg follicle begins to mature in response to rising levels of oestrogen, progesterone, follicle stimulating hormone (FSH) and luteinising hormone (LH). This occurs over an average of 10-14 days. Obviously its length may be variable. So the oestrogen acts to build up the uterine lining in preparation for the implantation of a fertilized egg. When the LH and FSH peak, a mature egg is released and this is called ovulation. Following ovulation, the luteal or the secretory phase begins. This is when the corpus luteum, the area on the ovary that used to house the egg, begins to secrete large amounts of progesterone. This stage lasts for another 14 days and is relatively constant.

The progesterone acts to keep the endometrial-lining stable in case of fertilization and implantation. If no fertilization occurs, the corpus luteum will stop functioning and endometrial shedding will occur, resulting in a menstrual period. This is a very simplified overview of what is going on. Organs that are involved in this process include the hypothalamus and the pituitary gland and the ovary. There is a complex interaction between these glands and the hormones, as described fully in the chapter on the endocrine system.

TERMS

One of the important things to do in this area is to be sure of your terms. Both the allopathic and homœopathic literature is full of arcane terms and it is well to know what they are talking about. So here goes with a quick whizz through some of the more common terms:

LEUCORRHOEA

This means discharge, usually outside of the usual menstrual discharge (although not uniquely).

LOCHIA

Is discharge after childbirth.

DYSMENORRHOEA

Means painful periods.

METORRHAGIA

Means bleeding between periods.

AMENORRHOEA

Absence of periods.

CLIMAXIS

Menopause by another name.

So…let's look at the most common problems and some of the associated factors:

FERTILITY, PREGANACY AND CHILDBIRTH

These are huge topics that require extensive specialist study in their own right and are not within the scope of this book.

ORGAN PATHOLOGY

ENDOMETRIOSIS

Endometriosis is a disease in which patches of endometrial tissue (which is, of course, usually found in the lining of the uterus – hence endometrium) grows somewhere outside of the uterus. This condition is seen most commonly in childless women between 30 and 40 years of age. The disease has no known predisposing factors – i.e. there's no known cause.

Usually endometriosis is confined to the lining of the abdominal cavity or the surface of the abdominal organs. The mislocated endometrial tissue commonly adheres to the ovaries and the ligaments that support the uterus. Sometimes though it adheres to the outer surface of the small and large intestines, the ureters, the bladder, the vagina, or surgical scars in the abdomen. It can even locate to the lining of the chest cavity and, rarely, the lungs. Because the misplaced endometrial tissue responds to the same hormones that the uterus responds to, it may bleed during the menstrual period causing 'chocolate cysts' in the ovaries as well as the expected (and associated) cramps, pain, irritation and formation of scar tissue. As the disease progresses adhesions occur and, of course, the misplaced endometrial tissue can interfere with normal functioning of the organ it has 'relocated' to. In rare circumstances (for example) adhesions can block the intestine.

DIAGNOSIS

Diagnosis of misplaced endometrial tissue can only be made if patches of endometrial tissue are seen. Other procedures include ultrasound scans, barium enemas, computed tomography (CT), and magnetic resonance imaging (MRI). Also certain blood tests can detect markers such as elevated levels of the antigen CA-125.

SIGNS AND SYMPTOMS

Endometriosis can present with some or all of the following symptoms. It is worth remembering that even quite severe cases can be completely asymptomatic (these cases are revealed when unexplained infertility is investigated).

- Pain in lower abdomen and pelvic areas
- Menstrual irregularities (e.g. spotting before normal periods)
- Infertility
- Dyspareunia (painful sexual intercourse)
- Abdominal swelling
- Pain during bowel movements
- Rectal bleeding during menstruation
- Lower abdominal pains during urination
- Unexplained constipation
- Anaemia

Endometriosis shares several characteristics with other diseases and it is as well to be aware of this. It can be mistaken for Menorrhagia, Fibroids, Chronic Pelvic Infection, and cancer of the Cervix. As the latter is the most 'worrying' for patients I've compared the two syndromes in the table shown here:

Endometriosis	**Cancer of the Cervix**
Heavy periods.	Heavy periods.
Painful periods.	
Irregular periods.	Irregular periods. Unusual discharge from vagina. Bleeding after menopause.
Pain on intercourse.	Pain on intercourse.
Abdominal swelling.	Abdominal swelling in advanced cases.
Spotting between periods.	Spotting between periods.
Unexplained infertility.	
	Bleeding after intercourse.
PMS.	
Pelvic pain..	Pelvic pain in advanced stages.
Common when giving birth after 30. Painful bowel movements.	Common in women with many pregnancies.

It's worth looking in some detail at some of the more important remedies for endometriosis, and their differentials; the table overleaf may help you:

ENDOMITRIOSIS REMEDIES

Remedy	Apis	Cactus	Caulophyllum	Lachesis	Palladium
Pain	Stinging, burning. Pain in ovaries after sex. Heaviness in uterus.	Painful constriction around pelvis. Pulling pains in uterus. Screams out with pain.	Erratic pains; spasmodic and severe. Drawing pains in thighs. Pain in small of back.	Pressing, stitching pain. Genitals very sensitive - can't even bear the weight of a sheet.	Shooting, burning and bearing down pain.
Menses	Supressed. Sense of tightness as if menses were about to appear. Menses last a day or appear at intervals of one day.	Flow ceases when patient lies down. Early. Lumpy, painful clotting.	Too soon and too scanty. Blood very light. Congested feeling during menses. Weakness over entire body during flow.	Delayed, scanty, intermittent. Fainting spells during menses. Menses black, scanty, lumpy. All complaints > flow.	Copious. Menstrual discharge whilst nursing.
Digestive	Thirstless. Constipation during menses.	Loss of appetite. Diarrhoea in the morning.	Bitter vomiting before menses. Nausea before menses.	Diarrhoea before menses. Vomiting before menses.	Constipation with menses. Abdomen sore after menses.
Mental / Emotional	'Declares she is well.' Fidgety, busy, clumsy. Whining tearfulness. Indifference.	Extreme fear of death. Weeping before menses. Sadness during menses.	Nervous, excitable, hysterical, fretful women.	Talkative. Suspicious. Vivid imagination. Sarcastic.	Strong desire for approval.
Modalities	Pain <heat, >cold <hot drinks, <touch, <5 p.m. > cool open air, > sitting.	< lying on left, <11am or 11pm > sitting, > open air.	<suppressed menses, < open air, < evening. > warmth.	< during and after sleep, < slight touch or pressure. > open air, > discharge.	<emotions, < standing, > touch and pressure, > lying on left side.
Con-comitants	Menses copious and lumpy with great pain in spleen.	Heart disease. Haemorrhage.	Joint pains with menstrual disorders.	Dysmenorrhoea pain shooting upward in left ovary on first day.	Nil
Worst affected	Heat of room or bed. Right side.	Left side.	Severe pain in small joints, especially carpal & metacarpal.	Left side.	Right ovary. Right side.
Key features	Scanty dark urine. Bearing down pains. Sharp, stabbing or plunging pains in uterus or in head. Enlargement of right ovary.	Severe dysmenorrhoea or metorrhagia with clots and constricting pain as each clot is passed.	Joint pains worse before menses > flow.	Profuse menses during climaxis. All aches relieved when flow starts.	Need for approval.

SALPINGITIS

Salpingitis – inflammation of the Fallopian tubes – occurs predominantly in women under the age of 35 who are sexually active, particularly with different partners. It is inflammation of the Fallopian tubes. This is usually the result of infection spreading upwards from the vagina through the uterine cervix and uterus and is commonly the result of inadequately treated primary infection, such as Chlamydia or gonorrhoea.

Other precipitating causes include interuterine devices (IUD) or complications following a termination of pregnancy. These infections very rarely occur before the first period, after menopause or during pregnancy. The infections are most commonly acquired during intercourse, although less commonly bacteria move into the fallopian tubes during a vaginal delivery or miscarriage.

DIAGNOSIS

This is suggested by the symptoms as well as an unusually high white blood cell count. Specimens are taken from the cervix and sometimes also from the rectum or throat. These are then cultured and examined for infective organisms. Occasionally conventional examination includes a needle inserted through the vaginal wall to obtain a pus sample.

SIGNS AND SYMPTOMS

Although symptoms may be worse on one side, both fallopian tubes are usually infected; this can spread into the abdominal cavity, causing peritonitis. The ovaries usually resist infection unless it is particularly severe – and the disease can be either chronic or acute.

The symptoms usually begin shortly after the period; chronic Salpingitis may follow on directly from an acute attack. Symptoms can include:

- Progressively severe pains in lower abdomen and pelvis
- Nausea or vomiting
- High fever with chills
- Tenderness of the abdomen (especially near the cervix)
- Irregular, usually heavy, bleeding
- Vaginal discharge
- Pain on intercourse
- Back pain
- General malaise
- Infertility

Salpingitis shares common symptoms with several other disorders, including: Appendicitis, ovarian cyst (especially in rupture), pyelonephritis (infection of the kidney), and ectopic pregnancy.

SALPINGITIS REMEDIES

Remedy	Apis	Eupion	Colocynth	Lachesis	Merc sol
Pain	Bearing down pains. Stinging pains in womb.	Burning, stinging. Itching and swelling between labia.	Severe vice-like cramping ovarian pain. Boring pain > doubling over. Dysmenorrhoea	Left sided ovary pain. Pain extends upwards. Pain > flow.	Colicky pain with exhaustion..
Menses	Severe dysmeno-rrhoea.	Period preceded by contracting pain and twisting in abdomen, followed by leucorrhoea and backache.	Suppressed after anger.	Dark, thick, clotted.	Milk in breast instead of menstrual flow.
Menstrual discharge	Scanty discharge of slimy blood.	Traces of menses between periods.	Coldness of hands and soles, rest of body is warm. Sweat at night. Sweat smells of urine.	Feet icy cold. Hot flushes. Sweat in axillae. Odour of garlic.	High fever and a severe toxic inflammation with sweating and exhaustion.
Fever	Fever with alternating sweats and dry heat.	Intense sweat from slightest exertion at night.	Nil	Copious fever; Smarting, staining and stiffening the linen.	Worse at night with itching and burning, smarting and soreness.
Leuco-rhoea	Profuse acrid green.	Copious dark (brown). Acrid and excoriating.	Nil	Greenish discharge.	Green leucorrhoea.
Modalities	< heat, touch, pressure. > cold, motion, sitting erect.	< during menses, cold. Pain in abdomen. > bending forward.	< emotions, lying on painless side, < night, < in bed. > hard pressure, > bending double, > heat, rest.	< after sleep, < morning, < heat, < slight pressure. > open air, > free secretions, > cold drinks.	< morning, < night, < lying down. > sitting up, > profuse diarrhoea.
Mental / Emotional	Weeping without cause.	Indisposed to talk during intermission of menses.	Impatient, easily angered.	Intense, goes to extremes. Strong minded, opinionated.	Irritability after eating. Morose after eating.

THRUSH

This is the common fungal yeast infection of the vaginal tract caused by the Candida albicans organism. Thrush can also affect other areas of mucous membrane, such as the inside of the mouth or indeed any moist skin. Infection in different areas may produce different symptoms.

The fungus that causes thrush is normally present in the vagina and the mouth. Its growth is kept under control by bacteria present in these organs. If antibiotic drugs destroy too many of these communal organisms, or if the body's resistance to infection is lowered (as in HIV & Aids) the fungus may multiply excessively.

Other factors that encourage the growth of Candida fungus include diabetes mellitus, hormonal changes during pregnancy, and the use of oral contraceptives.

Thrush can be contracted by sexual intercourse with an infected partner and is significantly more common in women than men.

SIGNS AND SYMPTOMS

Some patients may have Candidal infection and yet remain completely asymptomatic. The following is a list of some of the symptoms that may be manifested:

- Thick white discharge (commonly called 'cottage cheese' discharge)
- Curd-like deposits visible on the walls of the vagina
- Vaginal itching and irritation
- Discomfort passing urine
- Inflammation around the vulva and anal region
- Sense of urgency and frequency of urination
- Pain on intercourse
- Sensation of burning in the vagina with excess genital heat

DIAGNOSIS

Diagnosis is usually made through an examination of a sample of the white discharge, although, frankly, most women once diagnosed do not need to be tested again as they are perfectly capable of self-diagnosis.

There are a number of other conditions which can be mistaken for thrush, among them Chlamydia, cervical polyps, pelvic infection, gonorrhoea, and Trichomonas (a genus of parasitic flagellate protozoans which often infects the vagina). So it is worth making sure that the problem is exactly what you think it is. The latter is particularly difficult to differentiate from thrush as they both can have vaginal itching. Trichomonas is the 'milder' of the two – they both have burning in the vagina and pain on intercourse. The 'typical' discharge of the two differs in that Trichomonas has a greenish tinge and is frothy (where thrush is white and 'curd like'. If in doubt (as ever) send your patient off to the doctor for appropriate investigation.

THRUSH REMEDIES

Remedy	Alumina	Borax	Hamamelis	Kreosotum	Pulsatilla
Discharge	Thick, clear or white.	Thick gelatinous in consistency like 'clear egg white.	Metorrhagia occurring midway between periods with a passive flow.	Yellow, acrid, colour of green corn.	Watery but variable yellow-green which can sometimes be clear and white.
Pain or itch	Intolerable itching without eruption.	Pain in back as if a hot iron were thrust through the lower vertebrae.	Sore feeling and bearing down pain in back.	Burning irritation.	Painless.
Urinary symptoms	Must strain at stool in order to urinate.	Bladder pain on retaining urine.	Increased desire for urination. Irritation of the urethra followed by discharge and burning.	Involuntary urination at night. Frequent urging to urinate preceded by a white discharge from the vagina which stains clothes yellow.	Increased desire for urination. Burning of urethra during urination.
Genitalia	Leucorrhoea during the daytime only.	Leucorrhoea between menses.	Leucorrhoea with much relaxation of the vaginal walls.	Leucorrhoea with putrid, excoriating discharges and great itching. Swelling and excoration of the vulva.	Milky leucorrhoea with swelling of the labia.
Modalities	< In the morning on waking, < warmth. > evening.	< downward motion. > pressure, > 11 p.m.	< pressure, air, < motion. > rest.	< rest, < during menses. > warmth, > motion, rest, pressure.	< warmth, evening, < beginning motion, < lying. > cold, fresh open air, > rubbing, > lying on the back.
Sleep	Disturbed before menses.	Impossible on the right side. Sleeplessness after midnight.	Restless at night.	Dreams of urinating. Disturbed sleep. Great desire to sleep.	Sleeplessness from thoughts.
Mental / Emotional	Slowness in answering questions and vague replies.	Shrieking in sleep and starting from slight noises.	Exhaustion.	Frequent yawning.	Nil

DISORDERS OF MENSTRUATION

Ensure you are familiar with terms as covered on page 182.

DYSMENORRHOEA

One of the most important factors in treating dysmenorrhoea is to consider the aetiology, which can be summarised under a number of headings:

PSYCHOLOGICAL

Emotional symptoms can often precede dysmenorrhoea, such as conflict, grief, or (often) suppressed anger. What you need to do is to question very closely when the dysmenorrhoea started and what was going on at that time but also to consider the mental state during, or preceding the period. Are they angry, irritable, resentful, bitter and so forth. This mental state may be related to the emotions that were present at the beginning. Say they've had menstrual cramps for 10 years since age 23 and you can trace that state back to a bitter end to an important relationship at that time – the emotions can be a reliving of the anger, frustration, and grief from that time. This explains why so many cyclic emotions are seen by the patient (and especially the partner) as completely irrational. They are irrational in time, but only because they are frozen in time – at their aetiology they were the appropriate emotions.

Obviously, when you choose a remedy it doesn't matter how many physical particulars you take from the case, you'll only palliate if you can't find the remedy that the patient needed all that time ago when the problem started.

HORMONAL

The biggest issue in this aetiology (in that it occurs most frequently) is the birth control pill, which therefore needs careful scrutiny. Other hormonal factors to check are around states that are < since puberty, < since weaning a child, < since pregnancy. The remedy needs to be one that covers the dysmenorrhoea and also has a hormonal component.

INFECTION

This is another common aetiology. The periods have never been the same since…vaginitis, pelvic inflammatory disorder, oophoritis (inflammation of the ovaries), salpingitis and so on. If you perceive a suppression of discharges from infection, the remedies to consider (in this instance) would be the sycotic, particularly *Medorrhinum* and *Thuja*.

ALLERGIES

Patients who are allergic in general and/or who have allergic reactions often find that the allergy state is heightened with the onset of their periods. In this case you should be strongly considering a psoric remedy – one that has dysmenorrhoea and allergy states.

DRUGS AND TRAUMA

These are the other two main aetiologies – you don't need me to tell you to look for these, but I might need to remind you that dysmenorrhoea can be associated with something as simple as a localised trauma and that even long-standing and severe cases have been resolved with the 'usual suspect' remedies of *Arnica, Bellis, Ruta*, and so forth.

HOMŒOPATHIC TREATMENT

My top dozen remedies are listed below. Most homœopaths would have a different 'top list' (and mine changes now and then too). It is inevitable that, with such a common disorder, no list could be complete – however, this will be a good place to start:

COLOCYNTHIS

This has severe dysmenorrhoea with sharp stabbing pains. The keynote (the 'super-keynote', even) is that they have spasms, severe spasms and it doubles them over. They don't want to be touched, they don't want to be moved and they will cry and scream. So there's a clear picture of what she looks like; crying, screaming, and spasmed into a ball. The key modalities are that they are better for pressure and better for heat. These are the women who will go to bed with menstrual cramps; they want a hot water bottle that they press into the painful area, and her husband and children will know to leave her alone – if they know what's good for them.

MAGNESIUM PHOSPHATE

One of our tissue salts – the key differential for cramping is that *Colocynthis* tends towards the left and *Mag phos* tends to the right. Also Mag phos is better heat first and better pressure second, whereas *Colocynthis* is the reverse – the number one 'hot water bottle' remedy. But also happy in a hot bath!

DIOSCERIA VILLOSA

This is a yam, wild yam from Mexico and it is from this yam that hormones are extracted – so a lot of sexual hormones are found in it. It's going to be a big generative area remedy. Just like *Colocynthis* they have severe cramps and spasm in the uterus, but the keynote modality is that they are better for bending backwards – the opposite of *Colocynthis*. They arch their back – even in bed you'll see the difference in postures between these two remedies. They can have such severe cramping that it is manifest even in the fingers and toes (*Cuprum met*) – so when the uterus goes into spasm, so do their fingers and toes…so severely that they hurt.

BELLADONNA

So, with this remedy, (as usual) the idea is around the blood flow. All the blood flows to the uterus, it rushes there. So they will feel congested, hot, and may have a strong concomitant which will be…a fever. If they are in bed when you see them, just do the usual Belladonna trick of kicking the bed and see what the reaction is (<< Jarring). One of Kent's tricks was to wander in to the room and biff the bed – if the patient immediately aggravates, you're well on the way to a prescription. So…the usual *Belladonna* symptoms: hot, full feeling, often with a bearing down pain, the uterus feels heavy. Also look for the 'standard' flushed face of *Belladonna*.

CACTUS GRANDIFLORUS

Another instance of looking for the 'super-keynote' sensation of being constricted – not the word we use all the time when we're speaking English – but squeezing is what we normally say. "Like a hand has reached in and is squeezing the uterus, tighter and tighter". Even our older textbooks use this image 'as if an iron hand has grabbed the uterus and is squeezing it'.

CAULOPHYLUM

This is Blue Cohosh. It is an American Indian remedy for uterine problems – a great remedy for false labour pains, for tendency to miscarriage, for feeble labour and weakness in the uterus in general.

With dysmenorrhoea there is a bearing-down sensation and extreme exhaustion – so severe that the patient is wiped out for a couple of days. They can also be very chilly or perhaps have a chill – in that way they are similar to *Pulsatilla*.

This is one of the remedies that has an aetiology around the womb – so NBWS childbirth, or miscarriage, or abortion. Childbirth drains them and every month when the hormones change they get drained again and get cramps.

One of the remedies that is close to *Caulophylum* is *Gelsemium* – and they can quite easily be confused. They are both tired and weak and apathetic and suffer from general malaise; the differential is that *Gelsemium* is thirstless and *Caulophylum* is thirsty.

SABINA

This is particularly indicated in dysmenorrhoea with excessive haemorrhage of bright red blood and clots. The keynote for the pain is the location, which is from pubis to sacrum and it is a sharp pain. It is also one of the main remedies for women who are about to miscarry. And it can be used after childbirth in the case of bright red haemorrhage, especially with the characteristic pain. For comparison of this remedy look at *Thuja*.

IPECACUANHA

This is a Brazilian plant and in the local language Ipecacuanha means 'the plant that grows beside the road and if you eat it, it will make you vomit'… allegedly. So, if the patient has dysmenorrhoea with severe digestive problems, this may well be the indicated remedy. The key factors are dysmenorrhoea with bright red blood and vomiting or nausea.

Nux Vomica

Here we have one of the irritable remedies (You should be familiar with *Nux*, so I won't describe it too much) and like *Ipecac* they have what's called a toxic dysmenorrhoea – the digestive system is upset too. It feels as though they have a hangover – bilious, and ratty with headache and cramps. The 'super keynote' is the sensitivity…to noise and light and odours.

They are even sensitive to what they eat – many things giving them gas, or burning, heartburn, constipation, and so forth. This is the remedy where the children know most of all that mum should be left alone.

PULSATILLA

One of the main women's remedies anyway, so it's going to be a big one for dysmenorrhoea; this and *Sepia* are the big two. *Pulsatilla* has problems from the pill, menopause, hysterectomy, PMS, but the 'super-keynote' is the classic psychological picture that *Pulsatilla* displays. They feel abandoned, lonely, unloved, tearful. They will of course be better for consolation – you try to hug a *Colocynthis* and they will hit you – and *Nux* will throw something at you but *Pulsatilla* will ameliorate immediately. *Pulsatilla* is, as ever, better for walking outside in the fresh open air – even when they get chills with their cramps (which they do).

IGNATIA

This is where you find another remedy with a big psychological component. Dysmenorrhoea with a history of grief, dysmenorrhoea with 'conflict irresolution' and severe frustration. They may have a mild dysmenorrhoea every month, but if they have an argument with someone then the dysmenorrhoea is worse. They are hypersensitive like *Nux*, but it's a more hysterical type. It has more to do with mood changes – *Nux* has only one mood – ugly; *Ignatia* is changeable. They also sigh – "sits and sighs".

SEPIA

One of the classic dysmenorrhoea pictures; they have the usual bearing down pains, as if the whole uterus would drop out on the floor. So…. look for them having their legs crossed, or if they are holding themselves; as if to hold themselves in. There are similarities in this regard to *Belladonna*, but *Belladonna* has heat and *Sepia* is cold. They also have the standard PM backache with bearing down, unsurprisingly they are irritable and want to be left alone. Murphy says that this is the number one remedy for NBWS coming off the pill.

PRE-MENSTRUAL SYNDROME

Also known as pre-menstrual tension (and a host of other less flattering colloquialisms), this is a condition of nervousness, irritability, other emotional disturbances, and a range of physical concomitants. It is one of those diseases that are very difficult to describe precisely (it's very homœopathic in that everyone seems to be different) and yet pretty much everyone knows what it is.

SIGNS AND SYMPTOMS

- Water retention
- Mood changes
  - » irritability
  - » sadness & depression
  - » tearful
- Tenderness of the breasts
- Headaches
- Constipation
- Change of appetite – often a craving for chocolate
- Pains
- Sensation of uterine/pelvic congestion
- Skin problems – acne, cold sores
- Vaginitis
- Changes in libido
- For many of our patients PMS will be the main presenting complaint. For many more it will be an issue – just not the main one. For better or worse homœopathy has a good reputation for dealing with PMS and so you will see many, many patients with this syndrome. So here's a few remedies which may be of help – this is not an exhaustive list, just some of the more common ones and a couple of 'smaller' remedies:

AMBRA GRISEA

This remedy has hypersensitivity of the whole nervous system – so they may become even more sensitive premenstrually. This is something to bear in mind with all your patients; any pathology or 'area of affinity' is likely to be heightened by the imminent arrival of a period.

Ambra grisea people are sensitive at all levels, but are particularly vulnerable to being offended or criticised. This is the woman whose feelings are easily hurt, an unkind word will wound particularly at this time.

CALCAREA CARBONICA

Insomnia – especially premenstrually. *Calc carb* has ailments from anticipation – and this is something to anticipate (with anxiety, fear, dread, etc.) every month; and to lose sleep over. This is another remedy that is emotionally sensitive – sad music or movies will affect them.

Physically they suffer from cramps (in the feet and legs particularly) and oedema, specifically swelling of the breasts, which then get tender and sore.

CONIUM

This is a particularly good remedy for lumps in the breasts premenstrually, (or indeed at any time), they can be sad before their period with what is described in the literature as 'hints of irritability'.

Ignatia

Here's a classic remedy for mood changes, frustration and being argumentative. It is said to be indicated for women who are 'looking for a fight'.

Physically the sensitivity of the remedy is reflected in sensitivity to smells – they may especially not be able to tolerate strong perfume and/or cigarette smoke.

LACHESIS

This remedy gets manic before the period. They can become jealous (or more so) violent, abusive, and highly loquacious.

Physically they may have raised blood pressure, and the 'super-keynote' of the remedy is that everything is better (i.e. all their complaints, physical, mental and emotional) as soon as the flow starts.

LYCOPODIUM

This remedy is often thought of as predominantly male (which is probably true) but it is invaluable for women too. *Lycopodium* women find it difficult to make decisions premenstrually. They have a fear of making mistakes, and lack confidence "something is bound to go wrong".

Physically she may be bloated, flatulent, and have a strong craving for ice cream or chocolates.

NATRUM MUR

Most homœopaths would agree that this is another classic support remedy for PMS. This is well indicated for women who get very sentimental, they will listen to sad and moving music (preferably on their own) and get weepy. They can also be irritable and a little depressed and may "dwell on past disagreeable events". This is also one of the 'clumsy' remedies. Premenstrually they drop things and lose their balance.

Physically they crave salty food, crisps, nuts and such-like, and cheese. It is a remedy often used for headaches, especially premenstrually.

PULSATILLA

The patient who will benefit from *Pulsatilla* will usually be weepy, sad, suffer from oedema, and feel abandoned – "I'm all alone". They want to be held, and consoled and crave creamy foods.

SEPIA

There are homœopaths who would suggest that this is the number one remedy for PMS. Certainly it has been invaluable in many cases. These patients are irritable, depressed, have a lowered libido and are averse to consolation – "leave me alone!"

It is a remedy for women who are exhausted (and more so premenstrually) and who suffer from heaviness, especially in the pelvic region. It feels as if everything is 'bearing down'.

MENOPAUSE

Although the menopause is not a condition that practitioners are called upon to *cure* it is very common to see women in clinic for whom symptoms associated with the menopause form the major presenting complaints.

The main physical effect of the menopause is a greatly reduced production of oestrogen; the most commonly reported symptoms include:

- Hot flushes
- Night sweats
- Headaches
- Weight gain
- Insomnia
- Vaginal dryness

Naturally, as the menopause, marks such a significant change for women, it's not unusual for there to be psychological alterations too. Changes in the mental state can include irritability, sadness (even to depression), loss of mental acuity and a general apathy.

CONVENTIONAL TREATMENT

Not surprisingly the conventional approach most frequently used involves replacing the lost hormones....the cunningly named Hormone Replacement Therapy (HRT). This means that either oestrogen-only or a combination of progesterone and oestrogen is used to reduce the presenting symptoms.

The use of HRT remains contentious, as there are well-publicised damaging side effects (including increased risk of breast cancer and heart disease), but the fact remains that HRT remains popular even with patients also using homœopathic remedies. My experience has been that well indicated remedies can reduce (and even eliminate) the main presenting complaints even whilst the patient is on HRT, thus removing the need for the conventional medication.

HOMŒOPATHIC REMEDIES

It seems to me that there are a number of 'quick fix' remedies that will help in the short term with the most pressing symptoms….a few are listed below, but by far and away the most effective response seems to be good constitutional treatment. Often remedies that have been particularly resonant in the past for a patient will have a powerful action at this (and other) times of major life change.

That said – I have found these remedies to be a good starting place:

GRAPHITES

Where there is despondency and a general 'weariness' and a tendency to tears, and a noticeable loss of libido.

LACHESIS

I have found this to be immensely useful for hot flushes, both prophylactically and as an acute. It is also one of the very best remedies for headaches that are clearly associated with the menopause.

PSORINUM

Where the menopause has induced a deep (even suicidal) depression and/or when it is associated with a change in the skin tone – spots, pimples, rashes, and so on.

PULSATILLA

When the patient has become uncontrollably tearful and sad. Also indicated in insomnia and consequent tiredness, which causes the patient to be very sleepy during the afternoon, but then restless at night again.

SEPIA

Possibly the number one remedy choice of most homœopaths. Where there are significant changes to the psyche – patient becomes irritable and/or sad, rude to their family and very anxious. A great remedy for hot flushes and dryness of the vagina

ADJUNCTIVE TREATMENT

In my experience it seems that Vitamins C (500 – 1000mg) and E (800 IUs) taken daily can greatly help with hot flushes as can a decrease in dairy, caffeine, sweets and (rather obviously) alcohol.

In general I would advise gentle regular exercise eating smaller meals but more frequently. I have also found that women who take up (or return to) regular Yoga exercise have a much smoother passage through the menopause.

FURTHER READING

James Compton Burnett **Organ Diseases of Women**
B Jain Publishers
ISBN 81-7021-362-2

O A Julian **Materia Medica of New Homœopathic Remedies**
Beaconsfield Publishers
ISBN 0-906584-11-6

Dr Trevor Smith **A Woman's Guide to Homœopathic Medicine**
Thorsons Publishing Group
ISBN 0-7225-0842-5

Dr Dorothy Shepherd **A Physician's Posy**
C W Daniel Company Ltd.
ISBN 0-85207-272-4

Susan Curtis **Understanding Menopause - Natural Solutions that Really Work**
Neal's Yard Press (an imprint of Winter Press)
ISBN 9781905830053

Belinda Barnes **Preparing for Preganancy - The Foresight Programme**
Neal's Yard Press (an imprint of Winter Press)
ISBN 9781905830213

Miranda Castro
Homeopathy for Pregnancy, Birth, and Your Baby's First Year
St Martins Press
ISBN 0-312-08809-4 **www.gentlebirth.org**

NOTES

NOTES

CONTENTS

THE SKIN

As you know, the skin is there to keep the inside in, and the outside out. Without it all the bits and bobs in our body would drop out all over the carpet. Aside from this valuable role though, this impervious membrane constitutes a complete organ in and of itself. Indeed it is the largest organ in the body weighing about six pounds, and it performs a number of functions as detailed below:

- Regulation of the overall body temperature, as well as insulation
- Protection of the body from potentially harmful rays of the sun
- Manufacture and storage of vitamin D
- Elimination of unwanted substances
- Sensation of both painful and pleasant stimulation

Throughout the body, the skin's characteristics vary with respect to thickness, colour and texture. The head, for example, contains more hair follicles than anywhere else, while the soles of the feet contain none. In addition, the soles of the feet and the palms of the hands have much thicker layers.

Definitions for the skin
Stratifed simply means layered, and epithelium refers to surface tissue – the epidermis therefore is a layered tissue that 'sits' on the surface.
Sebum is an oily substance secreted by the sebaceous glands – it reaches the skin's surface through small ducts leading into the hair follicles. Sebum provides a thin layer of fat over the skin, and this serves two main functions – it slows the evaporation of water and has an antibacterial effect.

EPIDERMIS

The skin is composed of (essentially) two types of tissue – the epidermis, which forms the surface, and the underlying dermis. The epidermis is stratified epithelium.

The epidermis protects the body against friction, against loss of fluids and entry of germs. The pigmentation present in the epidermis shields deeper tissues against ultra violet light.

DERMIS

The dermis connects the epidermis to the underlying structures. It is made of tough, elastic connective tissue dense with nerves and blood vessels. The dermis is the layer that contains the different types of nerve endings for sensing temperature, pressure and, of course, pain. It is also in this layer that the sweat glands are situated; these are a major part of the body's cooling system, as well as the sebaceous glands that release sebum. Finally, this layer is rich in white blood cells that help to keep the skin clear of infections.

SUBCUTANEOUS LAYER

Beneath the dermis is a subcutaneous layer; this is looser connective tissue laden with fat deposits – it is this layer that gives a great deal of the body's insulation and to some extent acts as storage and padding.

PATHOLOGY

In the main, pathology of the skin is not life threatening, indeed often not even considered very serious. However, one should never underestimate the effect that a purely 'cosmetic' problem can have on a patient. Even the smallest blemishes can radically alter the way that someone views themselves and the manner in which they react to the world. Often skin problems cause anxieties around self-worth; these anxieties mean that the person's social interactions and skills are less effective. This in turn means that those around them will react less 'favourably', thus confirming any feelings of inadequacy. As practitioners we will often receive our most glowing testimonials from patients whose skin complaints have been eradicated – and consequently see a whole slew of new patients.

ECZEMA

So, let's start as usual with a definition. The term eczema means literally "to boil over" – which is a good description of the irritation and redness associated with the disease.

My medical dictionary defines eczema as a "superficial inflammation of the skin, mainly affecting the epidermis". Great. We know, of course, that eczema is usually characterised by redness and itchiness. Often we see small blisters that sometimes weep and/or become crusted. In practice we often see the nasty end of eczema in which the skin may scale, thicken, or discolour.

The label eczema covers a multitude of sins; the disorder has several forms, with two major divisions; **eczematous dermatitis** which is said to arise from external factors, and **endogenous eczema**, which is said to be constitutional. As homœopaths of course these label are of no use to us, but now at least you know what they mean. Characterisation of endogenous eczema is based upon its appearance and site as shown in the table below.

Diagnosis	Characteristics
Atopic	Commonly found in childhood and associated with a family history of allergy. Often the family history has hayfever and/or asthma, this may not mean much to our colleagues in the medical profession, but is vital for us homœopaths. Commonly found in the folds of the elbows and knees and therefore known as flexoral eczema.
Discoid	Small, well defined areas of eczema.

Seborrhoeic	Scaly plaques occur in areas of great sebum production. Sebum is the oily substance secreted by the sebaceous glands, which provides a thin, oily film of fat over the skin. This layer slows down the evaporation of water and acts as an antibacterial agent. Consequently seborrhoeic eczema is found most commonly at the site of greatest sebum production; the scalp, face, etc.
Varicose	Appears on the legs and is associated with poor circulation.
Pompholyx	Found on hands and feet. Pompholyx are unruptured vesicles that look like rice grains. They occur on hands and feet (in association with eczema) because the skin layer there is thick. (The greek word Pompos = bubble.)

CONVENTIONAL TREATMENT

Conventional treatment can appear successful, possibly due to the fact that, apart from the most severe cases, 90% of children with eczema will be symptom-free by the age of 10 (in fact Stephen Gascoigne says that girls will improve at 7 years and boys at 8 because these are the cycles in which we move). So it doesn't matter much what the doctors do, they will appear to be successful eventually in most cases. The start of eczema in children can be associated with vaccination or the introduction into their diet of cow's milk. Almost 50% of children who have eczema go on to develop asthma and/or hay fever. The more severe the eczema, the more likely the asthma is to appear.

If the eczema is not a childhood disease (and even if it is in some cases) the doctors will check for irritant substances (those which carry a risk of precipitating eczema) these include:

- Wool (due to lanolin, wool fat)
- Petroleum products and oils
- Cleaning agents
- Metals, eg. nickel in watches and jewellery
- Chemical used in deodorants, sprays and perfumes
- 'Biological' washing powders, detergents, soaps, etc.
- Rubber

Other important predicating factors may be found in the diet. This is particularly true of dairy products and of food additives. Eczema also has a strong hereditary component and if both parents had it, then the child has a 60% chance of developing it.

Apart from the advantage bestowed upon it by time, conventional treatment in reality, is not spectacularly successful. At best it can be said to be variable. The drug of choice is usually one of the corticosteroids. These can effectively suppress and mask the skin symptoms. Corticosteroids come in four potency levels as shown below:

Potency	Examples
Mild	Alcomethasone, Fluocinolone, Hydrocortisone, Methylprednisolone.
Moderate	Clobetasone, Desoxymethasone, Fluocinolone, Fluocortolone. Flurandrelone.
Potent	Beclomethasone, Betamethasone, Budesonide.
Very potent	Clobetasol, Diflucortolone, Halcinonide.

The use of corticosteroids leads (sadly) to an increased risk of infection or sudden spreading of skin symptoms if an infection is already present. Consequently there are a number of applications which are a combination of corticosteroid and antibacterial or anti-fungal agent. Unfortunately the application of these agents (as well as being suppressive) is associated with a high risk of allergic reaction. This will result in a condition (and symptoms) which are identical to the original condition. Brilliant!

HOMŒOPATHIC TREATMENT

Treating eczema can go one of two ways, frankly. You can immediately eradicate the evil rash from the babe in arms and be hailed as a miracle worker. Or you can spend several months trying to cure it. It has to be said that experience helps, and there are homœopaths who do particularly well with eczema. We all get a lot of cases; it is practically epidemic (or should that be pandemic?). And personal reputations can be made (or lost) on the treatment of eczema. So let's look at some remedies and their use by 'place'. Don't forget that there's no substitute for a properly prescribed constitutional remedy. That said, of course, here are some interesting differentials:

Remedy	Differentials
Antimonium crud	Particularly useful for eczema of the face and genitals.
Bovista	For the back of the hands.
Cicuta	For the chin.
Graphites	Eczema of the palms.
Mezereum	Eczema of the scalp with a lot of exudates.
Petroleum	Eczema, which cracks easily, especially behind the ears.

As I said, this is going to be a really big component of all clinics, so to give you a top notch chance of finding a suitable remedy here's another table. These are just a few of my favourite remedies with hints on each of them.

Remedy	Characteristics	Sensation	Modalities
Alumina	This is a dry remedy, with dry, thickened skin and deep, bloody cracks.	Itching < warmth. Burning < scratching.	Chilly < warmth, < dryness. >damp, < morning.
Arsenicum	Associated with restlessness and anxiety. Dry and scaly skin.	Itching > warmth. They scratch until it bleeds. Feels like worms under the skin	< undressing. Chilly > warmth. < 12-3 a.m. Periodicity.
Berberis	Is a first rate kidney remedy – so if there's a kidney function element this is a good choice.	Burning itch which wanders and is worse for scratching. Bubbling sensation. Numbness.	Left sided remedy. < dark. Also < night time. Radiating pains.
Graphites	One of the great skin remedies, characterised by honey-like discharge and deep bloody fissures.	Burning. Prickling. Wandering.	> open air, > on walking. < from suppression, < bright light. Desires beer.
Hepar sulph	An excellent 'acute' remedy for painful sensitive eruptions. The skin may appear unhealthy.	Sticking, splinter-like pains. A whole host of eruptions – pimples, scabs, vesicles, pustules.	< cold air. >warm air. < wool, < undressing, < draught.
Lycopodium	Associated with emotional aetiology. Eczema and gastric troubles.	Eruptions on perspiring parts. Crusty eruptions.	< evening, < on perspiring parts, < warmth.
Medorrhinum	Difficult to repertories, this is nonetheless a splendid remedy, especially for allergic eczema.	Fetid crusty eruptions, with a redness which remains after eruption has gone. Rubbing helps.	< evening and night. > rubbing gently. < thinking of it, < undressing.
Petroleum	Severe and distressing eczema with deep and bloody cracks. Terrible dryness.	Roughness – thick hard skin. Burning and smarting. Itching of orifices.	< night, < open air. > warmth. < travelling.
Psorinum	Eczema behind the ears. Dirty looking skin. Offensive discharges. Pus.	Itching. Itching even without eruption. Dryness – poor perspiration.	< cold air, <undressing, < wool. History of suppression.
Sulphur	The best-known skin remedy – has been known to cause aggravation before cure.	Itching and burning. Scratches until raw. Redness.	< warmth, < warmth of bed, < suppression. Hungry at 11 a.m.

Of course this is just a really quick *aide memoir* as there are dozens and dozens of remedies that might be suitable to treat eczema. It is highly likely that, at some stage, the patient will need a deep constitutional remedy along with more 'palliative' remedies to help the immediate distress. It is my experience that when treating children, one needs to be particularly attentive to the parents. Eczema can be as distressing for them as for the sufferer. Parents will often need careful education, clear prognosis, good lines of communication, and, frankly, a good remedy themselves.

DERMATITIS

This is an inflammation of the dermis and epidermis; usually in response to stimulation from trauma, temperature, chemicals, or food. If the skin inflames this is defined as dermatitis; if it swells up this is usually referred to as urticaria. In many circumstances dermatitis is used as an interchangeable definition with eczema. Strictly speaking though, eczema may have no observable aetiology whereas dermatitis does – examples include washing powders, bleach, animal fur, specific soaps, and so on. Symptoms include rashes, blisters, lesions, sores, and itching or cracked skin.

HOMŒOPATHIC REMEDIES FOR DERMATITIS

For our purposes we can usually treat with the same remedies that would be indicated for eczema. It might be worth remembering that *Chamomilla* can sometimes be really well indicated for children, and adults have responded well in acute situations to *Rhus tox*, *Mercury*, and *Silica*.

PSORIASIS

In the normal run of things, the epidermal cells are constantly being formed in the deepest layers and they 'migrate' to the outer layers of the skin to be finally shed at the surface. As they develop they are hardened by Keratin and this causes the cells to die.

Definitions for this page
Keratin is a fibrous protein that forms the body's horny tissues in a process called keratisation-the cells become flattened, lose their nuclei and fill with keratin.

In psoriasis the rate of keratisation is massively speeded up, so that the process (which should take a month or so) occurs in a matter of days. Consequently the process itself is inadequate, leading to cells sticking together. The skin thickens and has a silvery appearance and, inevitably flakes off prematurely leaving behind a reddish or pink patchy rash.

The disease affects roughly 2% – 4% of the white population, and there is a tendency for it to occur in the late teens and to improve with age; there is also a strong familial link. Although psora means 'the itch', it is not a particularly itchy disease.

CONVENTIONAL TREATMENT

As the disease is responsive to cyclosporine (an immunosuppressive drug) it is thought that the primary factor of the pathology may be immunological. Nonetheless the first choice in treating psoriasis is usually topical. Lubricating creams such as white petrolatum are often used – sometimes alone and sometimes in conjunction with topical corticosteroids. Ultraviolet B light is also an option. In extremis oral methotrixate is used, but as this is usually used as part of an anticancer regime (chemotherapy) this would probably be a last resort.

HOMŒOPATHIC TREATMENT OF PSORIASIS

It is important to consider the influence that inheritance plays in this disease (as in many diseases in fact) and try to tailor remedies to those factors as well as trying to find something to ease the problems as quickly and effectively as possible. See the table below and overleaf for ideas; I have used some of the lesser remedies rather than repeat the 'usual suspects'.

Remedy	Characteristics	Modalities
Arsenicum iodatum	Marked exfoliation of the skin in large scales leaving a raw surface below. Possible exudates – persistently irritating and corrosive. Night sweats.	< night. > open air. < exertion < tobacco smoke.
Clematis erecta	This is more likely to itch than one would expect, worse area around the scalp and occiput. Red and burning vesicles.	< washing in cold water. > perspiration. < heat of bed.
Manganum aceticum	Worse around the joints, especially the bends of the elbows and knees. Burning sensation.	> eating, swallowing, > open air. < touch < at night.
Mezereum	History of eruptions, which ooze acrid and gluey liquid. Formation of thick crusts with either scabs or pus underneath.	> wrapping up < at night < heat of fire or bed. Also < cold air and draughts.
Nitric acid	It is likely that the location will be at, or near mucocutaneous orifices (that's where the outside meets the inside of the body.) Skin dry, eroded and cracked, especially in the bends.	< jarring, motion < milk or fatty foods, < cold air and dampness < evening and night time.
Phytolacca	Useful in the early stages of skin diseases. Skin is very dry and shrivelled. History of boils.	> warmth and dry weather > lying on the stomach < cold nights < motion < hot drinks.

Continues over...

Remedy	Characteristics	Modalities
Sepia	Blotchy skin, raw and cracked – as with other remedies, likely to be worse in the flexures. Thick crusts on the elbows. Offensive odour of the skin.	< after sex < pre menses < falling asleep < rubbing and scratching.
Staphysagria	Staphysagria patients get itchy, then they scratch the affected area, then the location of the itch changes. The skin can be strongly affected, but this pathology often alternates with joint pains.	> from sex < from anger and indignation < loss of fluids < tobacco

ACNE

Acne usually commences at or around puberty, when a surge of hormones triggers an increase in the activity of the sebaceous glands, which secrete sebum via hair follicles. The hair, sebum, and keratinocytes that fill the narrow follicle may produce a plug, which is an early sign of acne. The plug inevitably prevents sebum from reaching the surface of the skin through a pore; its natural route.

The mixture of oil and cells allows bacteria that normally live on the skin to grow in the plugged follicles. These bacteria produce chemicals and enzymes and attract white blood cells that cause inflammation. When the wall of the plugged follicle breaks down, it spills everything into the nearby skin—sebum, shed skin cells, and bacteria, leading to lesions or pimples.

SIGNS AND SYMPTOMS

Acne is often worse in winter and generally improved in summer – probably due to the beneficial effects of sunlight. Blackheads or whiteheads usually form and the skin can look inflamed. If the acne is particularly deep and inflamed there can be scarring.

TREATMENT

Conventionally it is said that diet has little effect on acne, although this is not my experience, I would suggest that many adolescents do not pay much attention to their diet and an increase in fruit and vegetables (or maybe just a reduction in 'junk food') along with an increase in water intake can prove highly beneficial. Whether this is a direct result or simply that good diet better regulates rampant hormones is a moot point.

Good remedies include *Folliculinum* (for both males and females) a triad of '*Carbo*'s' – *Carbo veg, Carbo animalis, Carboneum sulph* and, of course *Psorinum* or *Sulphur*.

WARTS

Warts are a reaction of the epidermis to a virus (indeed they can be caused by at least 60 types of human papillomavirus). They can appear at any age but are most common in older children and less common in the elderly. Appearance and size of warts will often be dependant on location and on the amount of irritation and consequent trauma.

CONVENTIONAL TREATMENT

Many conventional practitioners take the view that warts will, if left alone, go away of their own accord. If they or the patient are in a hurry to get rid of them, however, the initial approach will usually be with topical acid based solutions or freezing with liquid nitrogen.

HOMŒOPATHIC TREATMENT

It is very common that *Thuja* is the main remedy of choice. It can be used in low potency, high potency, or even crude in tincture form (applied to the wart). If *Thuja* proves ineffective I'd be inclined to check out some of the homœopathic acids – notably *Acetic acid, Benzoicum acid, Fluoric acid, Nitric acid* or *Oxalic acid.*

FURTHER READING

Robin Logan **The Homœopathic Treatment of Eczema**
Beaconsfield Press
ISBN 0-906584-47-7

Robin Hayfield **Homeopathy for Common Ailments**
Gaia Books
ISBN 1-85675-021-3

Dr Dorothy Shepherd **Homœopathy in Epidemic Diseases**
Health Science Press
ISBN 0-85032-185-9

H A Roberts **Boenninghausen's Therapeutic Pocket Book**
B Jain Publisher
ISBN 81-7021-010-0

Joni Loughran **Natural Skin Care**
B Jain Publishers
ISBN 81-7021-995-1

Adrianna Holman **Understanding Eczema - Natural Solutions that Really Work**
Neal's Yard Press (an imprint of Winter Press)
ISBN 9781905830022

NOTES

NOTES

CONTENTS

MENTAL HEALTH

The treatment of mental illness is well established in this country. The oldest institution in the British Isles is the monarchy. The second oldest is a mental hospital (actually the original Bedlam, now the Bethlem Royal Hospital). There is a long and chequered history of psychiatric care in the UK and I hope to show that homœopathy has its place in the future care of the mentally ill, and that it need not be too daunting a task.

DEFINITIONS

Mental illness is defined as "psychological and behavioural syndromes that deviate significantly from those typical of human beings enjoying good mental health". This is a bit like saying good health is that which we have when we're not ill. There's no arguing with the exactitude of the definition; it just doesn't tell us much. In general we know that a mental disorder involves distress or impairment in important areas of functioning. But again this isn't always true. Some people can be quite mentally ill and still function relatively normally and with little or no distress.

For the greater part of recorded history, mental deviations were considered supernaturally or unnaturally caused, the work of evil spirits or human depravity. There is still a belief in some areas that mental illness is something supernatural.

After small beginnings in the 16th and 17th centuries, however, the science that eventually developed into psychiatry acquired respectability in the 1790s. At that time the Parisian physician Philippe Pinel abolished physical restraints, introduced moral (psychological) treatment, and began objective clinical studies; although this did not spread universally even into the 20th century.

CLASSIFICATION

The division of mental disorders into classes is still inexact, and classification varies from country to country. For official record-keeping purposes, most countries follow the International Classification of Diseases of the World Health Organisation (WHO). In its relatively short history the International Classification of Diseases system has undergone a number of revisions. It is now on its ninth revision, known as ICD-9. This may be telling us something about the exactitude of classification.

The other great work on classification has been distilled into the Diagnostic and Statistical Manual. This work is prepared and published by that august body, the American Psychiatric Association. It was first published in 1952 and was revised in 1968 and 1980. Again a sign that classification is not an exact science.

Furthermore, according to recent texts the "actual usage lags behind the mandated nomenclature" – meaning that they're not using the words that we're using. For example, the latest version (DSM- III) no longer has any classification of neurosis (they use the term disorder), although there's hardly a textbook in psychology that doesn't use the word neurosis.

It is only in the later versions of the DSM that homosexuality is no longer regarded as a psychological disorder in and of itself.

MENTAL HEALTH IN CHILDREN

Most classification systems recognise childhood disorders as separate categories from adult disorders, and the following represent a small but typical selection seen in clinic.

SPECIAL NEEDS

These patients are characterised by the inability to learn normally and to become as independent and socially responsible as others of the same age in the same culture. In homœopathic clinics it is more likely that we will come across children whose needs are specifically educational (rather than social), and certainly homœopathic remedies can help those children.

Remedy	Comments
Calcarea carbonica	Possible first choice. Slow, forgetful, obstinate. Mental effort produces a hot head. Averse to work or exertion. < exertion, < cold, < full moon, > dry climate, > lying on painful side, > sneezing.
Baryta carbonica	Either joint first or close second choice. Backward children, mentally and/or physically weak, low confidence. Bashful, confused. < thinking of illness. > walking in open air.
Agaricus	Confusion, disinclination to work, depression. < open air, > moving about slowly.
Lycopodium	Averse to starting new things, apprehensive, spells or writes wrong words. < heat, > getting cold.
Mercury	Slow in answering questions, weak memory and loss of willpower. < night, perspiration.

These remedies are (as ever) just suggestions and are the 'usual suspects' – it remains true that there is no substitute for a well-chosen constitutional remedy.

ATTENTION-DEFICIT HYPERACTIVITY DISORDER (ADHD)

This set of disorders includes conditions marked by inappropriate lack of attention, by impulsiveness, and by hyperactivity, in which the child has difficulty organising and completing work, is unable to stick to activities or follow instructions, and is excessively restless. This syndrome may be indicative of the tubercular or sycotic miasm.... so remedies to consider would be *Tuberculinum* and *Medorrhinum*.

PERVASIVE DEVELOPMENTAL DISORDERS

These are characterised by distortions in several psychological functions, such as attention, perception, reality testing, and motor movement. An example is infantile autism, a condition marked by unresponsiveness to other people, bizarre responses, and gross inability to communicate. Use the Repertory and look in the sections on

Mouth:

- » Speech,difficult
- » Speech, stammering
- » Speech unintelligible,
- » Speech, wanting

- Mind :
  - » Aphasia
  - » Forgetful of words
  - » Inability to articulate
- Children:
  - » Retarded mentally
  - » Idiocy
  - » Dyslexia
  - » Learning disabilities

...and so forth

ANXIETY DISORDERS IN CHILDREN

These include fear of leaving home and parents (separation), excessive shrinking from contact with strangers (avoidance), and excessive, unfocused worrying and fearful behaviour and many others. Anxiety disorders in children are becoming increasingly common. In general terms we can treat in the same way as anxiety states in adults – so we'll move on to that ...

ORGANIC MENTAL DISORDERS

This group of disorders is characterised by psychological or behavioural abnormalities associated with transient or permanent impairments in brain function. The disorders have different symptoms, depending on which area of the brain is affected and on the cause, progression, and duration of the disorder. Organic damage to the brain can result from a disease or drug that directly damages the brain, or from a disease that indirectly damages the brain through effects on other bodily systems.

Symptoms associated with organic mental disorders may be a direct result of organic damage or may be the patient's reaction to lost mental abilities. Some disorders have as their primary feature delirium, or a clouded state of consciousness, which is manifested by difficulties in sustaining attention, by sensory misperceptions, and by disordered thought.

Another common symptom, especially in organic mental disorders associated with old age, is dementia. Dementia is marked by impairments in memory, thinking, perception, judgment, and attention that are sufficient to interfere with social and occupational functioning. Emotional expression is also often changed, as evidenced by increased apathy, euphoria, or irritability.

ALZHEIMER'S DISEASE

Alzheimer's disease is covered fully in the Nervous system chapter.

SCHIZOPHRENIA

Schizophrenia is a group of serious disorders, beginning usually in adolescence or young adulthood. Symptoms include disturbances in thought, perception, emotion, and interpersonal relationships.

Once again this is not something that we would routinely expect to treat, although there is no reason why homœopathy should not help the sufferer. Certainly conventional treatment – usually major tranquillisers or ECT – is not amazingly successful, nor is it particularly pleasant. The most common of the major tranquillisers (and still frequently used) is Largactyl (Chlorpromazine in this country, Thorazine in the US).

It is called Largactyl because it has some of the largest actions of any drug upon the body. Amongst the side effects of Largactyl are:

- extrapyramidal symptoms (the shakes)
- tardive dyskinesia (rolling up of the eyes)
- hypothermia
- drowsiness
- apathy
- pallor
- nightmares
- insomnia

- depression
- nasal congestion
- dry mouth
- constipation
- hypotension
- tachycardia
- impotence
- weight gain
- photosensitisation
- rashes
- jaundice
- and many others

So it's difficult to believe that there's anything homœopathy (or any other complementary therapy) could do which would be worse. Largactyl does not cure schizophrenia to any notable degree; it simply makes the illness more bearable.

For an outstanding description of the 'feeling' of schizophrenia I would recommend the book 'Operators and Things, the inner life of a schizophrenic', by Barbara O'Brien (pub. Abacus Books) or spending some time in a psychiatric institution and talking to the patients there.

Schizophrenia has long been recognised as having a familial content, so this is likely to lead us to consider miasmatic remedies.

DELUSIONAL (PARANOID) DISORDERS

The central feature of the paranoid disorders is a person's delusion (a firmly held false belief), for instance that he or she is being persecuted or conspired against. In another form, the delusion consists of unreasonable jealousy. The person may be resentful, angry, sometimes violent, socially isolated, reclusive, and eccentric. The disorder usually starts in middle or late adult life and can be seriously disrupting to social and marital relationships.

NUTRITIONAL TREATMENT

According to Dr. Abram Hoffe, Canadian Director of Psychiatric Research tranquillisers "never cure mental illness because they replace one psychosis with another". He favours nutritional intervention, which, he says, cures 80% of acute schizophrenia (there are many differences between acute schizophrenia and chronic schizophrenia, but that's a whole other discussion). His definition of cure is threefold, it means that his patients:

- socialise with family and community
- are free from symptoms
- pay income tax

The latter criteria is important because patients on major tranquillisers do not usually hold down a job.

Early nutritional trials with niacin (vitamin B3) showed that niacin doubled the recovery rate from acute schizophrenia. This was in 1953! Because these results were not duplicated with chronic schizophrenics, interest in niacin therapy quickly died. Other trials have also shown that vitamin B6 can help schizophrenia.

Patrick Holford (author of many good books on the subject of nutrition, including 'The Optimum Nutrition Bible') recommends the following:

Cut out or avoid sugar and refined foods. Cut down on stimulants – tea, coffee, chocolate, cola, alcohol, cigarettes, and follow a healthy, sensible and balanced diet. Plus add in extra quantities of:

- Multivitamins
- 2 x Vitamin C 1000 mg
- Multimineral with
- zinc
- magnesium
- manganese
- chromium
- Extra folic acid (a B vitamin)

HOMŒOPATHIC TREATMENT

There are many homœopathic remedies that would help in treating schizophrenia. If nothing else, the remedies may help with some of the side-effects of the conventional medication. As usual…take the case. The Repertory is full of rubrics that may relate to the specific conditions of any individual's circumstances. Good ones to look at include:

- Insanity
- Mania
- Multiple personality
- Dementia
- and of course Schizophrenia

Remedies to consider would include *Aurum, Anacardium, Lachesis, Stramonium* and *Arsenicum*. It is likely that the predominant miasm will be syphilitic.

AFFECTIVE DISORDERS

The affective disorders are those in which the predominant symptom is a disturbance in mood. One form, depression, is marked by sadness, guilt, and feelings of helplessness and hopelessness. In mania, the mood is elevated, expansive, or irritable.

DEPRESSION

This is the psychiatric disorder characterised by feelings of worthlessness, guilt, sadness, helplessness, and hopelessness. In contrast to normal sadness or the grief accompanying the loss of a loved one, clinical depression is persistent and severe. It is accompanied by a variety of related symptoms, including disturbances in sleep and eating, loss of initiative, self-punishment, withdrawal and inactivity, and loss of pleasure.

Community surveys show that as many as 20 in 100 people suffer from significant depressive symptoms at any one time; some 25 percent of the population may suffer from a depression over the course of a lifetime. The disorder strikes men and women of all ages, in all segments of society, but most studies indicate that women are more often afflicted.

TYPES OF DEPRESSION

In psychiatry, two major forms of depressive disorders are recognised. In both, the predominant symptom is a disturbance in mood. One form of the disorder, depressive disorder, is marked only by episodes of depression. The other, bipolar or manic-depressive illness, is characterised by alternating depressed and manic episodes.

In major depression or the depressed phase of bipolar illness, a depressed mood predominates, although the patient may not be aware of feeling sad. Typically, he or she loses all interest in and withdraws from usual activities.

SIGNS AND SYMPTOMS

These include sleep disturbances (usually early-morning awakening), loss of appetite or greatly increased appetite, inability to concentrate or to make decisions, slowed thinking and decreased energy, feelings of worthlessness, guilt, hopelessness, and helplessness, diminished sexual interest, and recurrent thoughts of suicide and death, sometimes leading to actual suicide. In the manic phase of bipolar illness, the patient's mood can be elevated, expansive, or irritable. Behaviour is bizarre and sometimes obnoxious. Other symptoms include excessive talkativeness, racing thoughts, and grandiose ideas, greatly increased social, sexual, and work activity, distractibility, loss of judgment, and a decreased need for sleep.

OCCURRENCE

Both depressive and bipolar disorders run in families. Almost certainly, a predisposition to these disorders is genetically transmitted. Thus, the risk of a depressive disorder is greater in the families of depressive patients than in the population at large. The higher proportion of depression in women may be biologically induced. Because women in trouble are more likely to seek help than men, statistics reporting a higher incidence of depression among women than among men may be explained, at least in part, by an under-diagnosis of depression in men.

CONVENTIONAL TREATMENT

The depressive disorders are among the most frequently treated in psychiatry. The usual treatment in modern practice involves administration of a drug plus supportive psychotherapy (or drugs alone). Two major classes of drugs are used to treat depressive disorders: the tricyclic/tetracyclic antidepressants and the monoamine oxidase (MAO) inhibitors.

The latter requires a special diet because they interact with tryamine, which is found in cheeses, beer, wine, chicken livers, and other foods, and causes elevation of blood pressure. The tricyclic antidepressants require no special diet; common generic drugs in this class are amitriptyline, desipramine, doxepin, and imipramine. Lithium carbonate, a common mineral, is used to control the manic phase of manic-depressive illness. In smaller doses, it is also used to regulate the mood fluctuations of this bipolar disorder.

Electro-convulsive therapy, or ECT, is occasionally considered effective for depressions not responsive to drug therapy. Although controversial, ECT can sometimes bring rapid relief from severe depression and can often prevent suicide.

NUTRITIONAL TREATMENT

There are many nutritionally-related causes of depression; probably the most common is sub-optimum nutrition, which results in poor mental as well as poor physical energy. Disturbed blood sugar balance can result in periods of depression. Patients who produce excessive amounts of histamine are also prone to it. Similarly adrenal exhaustion brought on by stress or over-use of stimulants can have the same effect. It is also the case that allergies can cause depressive illness.

Advise your patients to experiment for a couple of weeks without any wheat or dairy products. As usual cut out or avoid sugar and refined foods. Cut down on stimulants – tea, coffee, chocolate, cola, alcohol, and cigarettes. And follow a healthy, sensible and balanced diet.

- A good multivitamin
- A Multimineral with at least
    - 10mg Zinc
    - 200mg Magnesium
    - 5mg Manganese
    - 100mcg Chromium
- 2 x Vit C 1000 mg
- Pantothenic acid 500 mg

HOMŒOPATHIC TREATMENT

There are innumerable homœopathic remedies and herbal remedies for depression, (one which finds favour in both camps at the moment is St. Johns Wort…Hypericum).

The main rubric for depression in the repertory fills nearly a full page (one of the largest in the book – what does this tell us?) and the sub-rubrics fill the next couple of pages.

The table shown below shows a few to consider, but it really does require careful consideration and almost certainly a constitutional remedy.

Remedy	Characteristics
Aurum	Under a black cloud and potentially suicidal.
Calc carb	For depression with various fears.
Natrum mur	Weeps while alone.
Pulsatilla	Can't fight and doesn't care who sees her weep.
Sulphur	Depressed to the point of not caring.

LESSER-USED REMEDIES

The remedies in the table above are the more common ones and have been highly successful in treating depression over many years. Nonetheless there are an awful lot of additional, lesser-used remedies that may help and it may be an idea to try and 'think laterally' about some of these:

ACONITE

This is a remedy that is easily dismissed as one of the 'first year, first aid' remedies. Nevertheless, for depression that has stress as a clear aetiology, this can be a valuable prescription. It's useful for depression following an illness or a massive use of energy, don't forget that depression can be an 'acute response' and this, as one of our great acute remedies, may be priceless. The remedy can be characterised by sadness and irritability with no affection for anyone and a disposition to quarrel and argue. I have occasionally seen *Sepia* prescribed when *Aconite* would have been a much better choice, especially if the keynote symptom 'ailments from fear or fright' is present.

CHAMOMILLA

Here is another remedy that is thought of primarily as an acute remedy, but I have seen it effective in depression. This patient who needs this remedy has a broken heart she (usually) is agitated, discouraged and tearful. And when she cries she howls – this is not a quiet tear shed in private, but a sustained, public weeping. This is also one of the remedies where depression and anger can co-exist; they can be quite aggressive (so beware).

GELSEMIUM

Yet another of the remedies that may be dismissed as 'first aid'. However, this is one of our great polychrest remedies and is black type for depression in Murphy's Repertory. They have depression of the spirit that leaves them feeling 'vacant' in the mind – we may hear them complain of being 'empty-headed'. This remedy too has an aggressive side, and they don't want to be spoken to. They can also be suicidal, they feel suicidal (preferred method – jumping out of a high window) and this makes them feel even more depressed. They can cry and cry, and they feel so worried that they don't want to be left alone. They're worried that they'll lose control of themselves and do something harmful if left alone.

PLATINA

This is a remedy that may prove useful for bi-polar disorder; they can suffer from depression or mania. In the depressive state they feel that they stand alone in the world, and this adds to their depression. They are tearful involuntarily, so they can't control their tears and they make 'loud cries for help'. This isn't likely to be a quiet 'in the corner' kind of depression. It is loud and highly visible. This is another remedy that doesn't want to be left alone, in the case of *Platina* it isn't that she fears she will harm herself, but that she will harm (by stabbing) her loved ones – her husband or children.

POST-NATAL DEPRESSION

It may be worth looking at this 'subset' of depression to get some sense of the sort of remedies that can be useful. I also want to focus a little more on an area of depressive illness that homœopaths are more likely to see in clinic.

Post-natal depression (or postpartum depression) is very common. Somewhere in the region of 1 in 10 women will have a period of depression following childbirth. One of the patient management issues is that of diagnosis. It's thought that between 40% and 80% of women get 'the blues' after childbirth anyway; so how can we differentiate between that and a clinical problem? To be frank, it is really a question of intensity and duration. A deep, long-lasting depression is probably a clinical problem rather than a 'passing phase'; also deep depression will usually have been conventionally diagnosed.

As practitioners we need to be aware that the time following childbirth is one during which the mother is particularly vulnerable emotionally (as well as physically, of course). It is a fact that psychiatric hospital admission is more likely to occur in women following childbirth than at any other time of life. Indeed some 80% of these admissions will receive a diagnosis of affective disorder (depression). Women who are affected this way post-natally are hundreds of times more likely than the general population to experience postpartum depression with their next child. Something we need to be acutely aware of at the next pregnancy.

For many conventional practitioners there are reservations about giving medication to nursing mothers, so homœopathy may be perceived by the parties involved as a genuine 'alternative' (rather than just 'complementary') approach. So let's have a look at some possible remedies:

SEPIA

This is a possible number one choice. The mother displays an aversion to the child, to the husband, and to the other family members. She may also be lacking in the 'mothering instinct', and consequently not inclined to breast-feed. They want to be left alone and are irritable, exhausted and drained. The pregnancy and birth has truly worn them out, and they may well be anaemic.

IGNATIA

This remedy is more likely to be needed for the first pregnancy. It is indicated for the mother who has taken great pains to plan her pregnancy and the birth. She may have been doing all the special exercises, negotiating with the midwives and her GP about having a home birth, she's chosen the music and the setting carefully and is anticipating a beautiful and spiritual experience. She has high expectations. Then the actual birth arrives and she is faced with extreme labour pains, complications, poor timing, unforeseen difficulties, maybe hospital admission and so forth. Then. after the birth she suffers "ailments from disappointment", she feels as though she has failcd. There may be no 'rational' cause for this feeling, the child is healthy, mother is well and so on, but she feels as though she wasn't the strong, calm, 'spiritual earth mother' that she wanted to be. Consequently she gets moody, depressed, irritable, and upset.

FERRUM MET

Depression and apathy following childbirth, this remedy has a real aversion to any work or effort. So it may be needed for the mother who, prior to the birth, was a real 'career woman'. Someone who had planned a swift return to a job that she had found highly fulfilling and a centrepiece of her life, and now she is completely disinterested in going back to work. There may also be a lack of interest in the baby, and in her surroundings. This is a classic remedy for loss of blood and consequent anaemia (as is China) with an 'easy flushing of the face'.

PULSATILLA

After the birth the mother is very tearful and depressed, she wants a great deal of consolation – indeed she can be quite demanding about it – and may need constant reassurance. She may be worried unnecessarily about the baby's health, or her own health, or the fidelity of the father, and will require repetitive reassurance that all is well.

Naturally with an area of pathology as large as this there are many, many potential remedies, but these few are a good place to start looking.

NEUROSES AND PSYCHOSIS

It is generally asserted that that the defining difference between neurosis and psychosis is that those afflicted with the former state have 'insight' into their condition.

Examples of neurotic disorders are those in which anxiety is the major symptom, hypochondriasis (morbid concern about health), panic attacks, phobias etc. It is true in very general terms the difference between neurosis and psychosis is that the psychotic patient lacks insight. Psychotic means, roughly, a state in which a patient has lost touch with reality, whereas neurotic refers to a relatively less impaired state. Schizophrenia, many organic mental disorders, and some forms of depression (such as manic-depressive illness) are psychotic conditions.

This is only a relatively useful distinction in terms of classification. It should be realised that it is an artificial distinction. It is not unusual for someone with a florid psychotic disorder ("I am the son of God", Napoleon, etc) to present themselves at a psychiatric institution rather than the more obvious place (like a church for example). If they had no insight (the classic distinction between psychosis and neurosis) they would not go to the hospital.

Again this is a somewhat flip assertion and doesn't always hold water. How many people do we know who do things which are not entirely rational but who have no insight into the degree of irrationality of their behaviour? (The partner in your life is usually a good target to find an example.)

Nonetheless, it is usually true in a clinical setting that patients with neurotic disorder have some degree of insight into their condition. Indeed they may often complain that they fear they are going mad. We know this to be a common fear, both empirically and because the rubric "Mind, fear, insanity of" is a relatively big one.

Neurosis in psychoanalytic terms is a mental illness characterised by anxiety and disturbances in one's personality.

Generally, only psychologists who adhere to a psychoanalytic or psychodynamic model of abnormal behaviour use the term *neurosis*. Psychiatrists and psychologists no longer accept the term as a formal diagnosis. Laypersons sometimes use the word *neurotic* to describe an emotionally unstable person.

In the psychoanalytic model, neurosis differs from psychosis, another general term used to describe mental illnesses. Individuals with neuroses can function at work and in social situations, whereas people with psychoses find it quite difficult to function adequately.

So it would be appropriate for us to look at anxiety states and to be aware that this is the study of neurosis. It also points us clearly to the area in the Repertory where we should start with our neurotic cases, namely in the Anxiety and Fears sections.

ANXIETY STATES

Anxiety is an emotional state in which people feel uneasy, apprehensive, or fearful. People usually experience anxiety about events they cannot control or predict, or about events that seem threatening or dangerous.

For example, students taking an important test may feel anxious because they cannot predict the test questions or feel certain of a good grade. People often use the words *fear* and *anxiety* to describe the same thing. Therefore, in practice it may be important to differentiate between the two, and if in doubt – use the patient's actual words. Fear also describes a reaction to immediate danger characterised by a strong desire to escape the situation.

The physical symptoms of anxiety reflect a chronic "readiness" to deal with some future threat. These symptoms may include fidgeting, muscle tension, sleeping problems and headaches. Higher levels of anxiety may produce such symptoms as rapid heartbeat, sweating, increased blood pressure, nausea, and dizziness.

All people experience anxiety to some degree. Most people feel anxious when faced with a new situation, such as a first date, or when trying to do something well; such as give a public speech. A mild to moderate amount of anxiety in these situations is normal and even beneficial. Anxiety can motivate people to prepare for an upcoming event and can help keep them focused on the task at hand.

In some senses homœopaths have an advantage in treating these (and other) psychiatric conditions in that we do not need to analyse or diagnose. Our Repertories are full of wonderful and precise descriptions of fears, delusions, anxieties, and so forth. To some degree homœopathy for the emotional condition requires no more (or less) skill than for the physical condition. It may however require a better 'bedside manner' or a different perspective, but that's a subject too wide for this book.

HOMŒOPATHIC TREATMENT

When treating anxiety states it is important to be aware of the *focus* of the anxiety and also any *concomitants* to the anxiety. Certainty about these two factors will greatly help in the search for a remedy. Here are a few differential conditions and remedies that may help in treating anxiety states:

ANXIETY THAT AN ACCIDENT MAY HAPPEN

This is a very common anxiety especially amongst new (or relatively new) mothers. The two main remedies are:

PHOSPHORUS

These are generally fearful people, afraid that something terrible lurks round every corner. They can be (or believe themselves to be) quite clairvoyant. They are easily troubled and greatly oversensitive to external impressions

MAGNESIA SULPHURICA

These are people who cry with anticipation – they are tearful *before* the event. They are almost beside themselves with worry and the focus can be others (the children, husband, etc.) or on themselves., they may fear that the accident will happen to them.

ANXIETY ON THEIR OWN

This is a very common anxiety state; people who are anxious just by virtue of being left on their own. They can't stand being alone. The big two remedies are *Arsenicum* and *Phosphorus*, remedies that are well known and well covered in other places, but it might be worth looking at some smaller remedies:

DROSERA

This is a well-known cough remedy, but it also has a big impact on anxiety states. These people imagine that people hate them, and they feel this especially when they are on their own. Their anxieties are magnified when they are alone. They are mistrustful and anxious, and especially they feel that those nearest and dearest to them are against them. They feel that they are unable to trust the very people that they should most be able to depend on.

MEZEREUM

This remedy suffers anguish, anxiety and restlessness when alone and they long for company. However, they don't make particularly good company – they are taciturn and indifferent. In company they can be peevish, slow and confused … not the ideal dinner party guest. So here is a remedy that places itself in the very situation they most fear.

PANIC ATTACKS

This is a very common anxiety state. One that will crop up again and again in the clinic. Good remedies are:

ACONITE

This is almost certainly the number one choice for panic attacks, when they are actually happening, and if they form a chronic condition. The attacks are accompanied by a fear of death and are likely to be a physical as well as an emotional experience – with palpitations, sudden increased perspiration, feeling faint and so forth.

ARGENTUM NIT

These are people who have been working at a hundred miles and hour – work, work, rush, rush, busy, busy, and then they go into overload and then … panic attacks. During the attacks there are changes of perception – especially related to time – and they can actually pass out.

KALI ARSENICUM

This is a very frightened and anxious remedy, so inevitably there is a possibility of panic attacks. These can then recur at regular intervals, maybe every third of fourth day. These patients are very, very nervous of *their panic attacks*. So what happens is that they may have one attack, at that's all it takes to add into their clinic picture 'fear of panic attacks'. Then the anxiety about the possibility of an attack (are you following this?) can lead them to have another attack. And the spiral is ratcheted up another notch.

I would caution that patients who have anxiety states as a major part of their presenting picture can sometimes be hard work. They may be demanding and can often be quite manipulative. It would be advisable in many instances for homœopathy to be one aspect of a multi-disciplinary approach, ideally including a reputable psychologist or behavioural psychotherapist. On the positive side my experience is that homœopathy can be wonderfully successful for patients who have found little or no relief along other routes.

FURTHER READING

Edward Whitmont **Psyche and Substance**
North Atlantic Books
ISBN 0-913028-66-5

Philip M Bailey MD **Homeopathic Psychology**
North Atlantic Books
ISBN 1-55643-099-X

Catherine R Coulter **Portraits of Homœopathic Medicines (Vols I – III)**
North Atlantic Books
ISBN 1-55643-036-1

Richard L Gregory (Editor) **The Oxford Companion to the Mind**
Oxford University Press
ISBN 0-19866-12-4-X

Dr Stephen gascoigne **Understanding Depression - Natural Solutions that Really Work**
Neal's Yard Press (an imprint of Winter Press)
ISBN 9781905830039

Richard Appignanesi **Freud for Beginners**
Writer and readers publishing cooperative
ISBN 0-906386-09-8

NOTES

NOTES

CONTENTS

THE VISUALSYSTEM

There is a strong psychological component to the visual process. We quite literally see what we expect to; so commonly accepted is this verity that there's a standard acronym – SET – 'See what we Expect To'.

This is something that was recognised as long ago as the seventeenth century; the philosopher Locke quotes a letter that he received from a colleague in which the problem was posed:-

"Suppose a man born blind, and now adult, (were) taught by his touch to distinguish between a sphere and a cube of the same metal and the same bigness. Suppose that the cube and the sphere placed on a table and the blind man made to see.... (could he) now distinguish and tell which were the globe and which the cube?" (Locke 1690)

Locke supported the empiricist view and concluded that the man would not be able to tell the sphere from the cube. We have since had a partial answer to this question from the studies of individuals who were born blind, and whose vision was restored in adulthood (Senden 1960). It transpires that when adults have the gift of sight for the first time they are confused by the bewildering array of visual stimuli. They were able to distinguish figures from the ground; they could fixate on figures, scan them, and follow moving figures with their eyes. So these abilities seem to be innate. However, the patients could not identify by sight alone many objects that were familiar by touch. They couldn't distinguish faces, knives, or keys. In addition they could not tell a triangle from a square (unless they hit on the cunning ruse of counting the number of corners or 'tracing' the outline with their fingers in an 'imitation' of touch). Further they couldn't tell which of two sticks was the longest without feeling them.

It took several weeks of training for these patients to be able to 'see' in the way that most of us take for granted. What we call sight, and generally consider a passive activity is in fact learned – we learn to see and sight is therefore an active process, not a passive one.

THE STRUCTURE OF THE EYE

The entire eye is a spherical structure approximately 2.5 cm (about 1 in) in diameter with a pronounced bulge on its forward surface. The outer part of the eye is composed of three layers of tissue. The outside layer is the sclera, a protective coating. It covers about five-sixths of the surface of the eye, continuous with the cornea at the front of the eyeball. The middle layer of the coating of the eye is the choroid, a vascular layer lining the posterior three-fifths of the eyeball. The choroid joins with the ciliary body and with the iris, which lies at the front of the eye. The innermost layer is the light-sensitive retina.

The cornea is a tough, five-layered membrane through which light is admitted to the interior of the eye. Behind the cornea is a chamber filled with clear, watery fluid, the aqueous humor, which separates the cornea from the crystalline lens. The lens itself is a flattened sphere constructed of a large number of transparent fibres arranged in layers; it is connected by ligaments to a ring-like muscle, called the ciliary muscle, which surrounds it. The ciliary muscle and its surrounding tissues form the ciliary body. This muscle, by flattening the lens or making it closer to spherical, changes its focal length.

EYE MOVEMENT

Six muscles that are directly attached to the eyeball control eye movements. The four rectus muscles form a relatively straight line from their points of origin, while the two oblique muscles approach the surface of the eye at an angle. All the muscles combine to keep the eyeball in nearly constant motion in order to maximize human vision, which is capable of focusing on about 100,000 distinct points in the visual field. These muscles also enable both eyes to focus on the same point simultaneously, thereby creating effective depth perception.

THE BONY BIT

The orbit, or eye socket, is formed by the juncture of a number of bones. Of these, the sections of the ethmoid bone are located between the orbits, forming part of the inner wall of each orbital cavity (called the orbital plate) and lateral wall and part of the roof of the nasal cavity. The frontal bone forms most of the upper surfaces, while the maxilla and malar (zygomatic) bone form the lower and outer surfaces. The lachrymal bone also forms part of the inner surface, in conjunction with the ethmoid bone.

SUMMARY

The eyeball lies nestled in fat within the orbital cavities of the skull, where it is situated above and lateral to the centre. Of all the senses, eyesight is often considered most important. According to one estimate, four-fifths of everything we know reaches the brain through our eyes. The eyes transmit constant streams of images to the brain by electrical signals. The eyes receive information from light rays. The light rays are either absorbed or reflected. Objects that absorb all of the light rays appear black, whereas those that reflect all the light rays appear white. Colored objects absorb certain parts of the light spectrum and reflect others. When you look at something, the light rays reflected from the object enter the eye. The light is refracted by the cornea and passes through the watery aqueous humor and pupil to the lens. The iris controls the amount of light entering the eye. Then the lens focuses the light through the vitreous humor onto the retina, forming an image in reverse and upside down. Light-sensitive cells in the retina transmit the image to the brain by electrical signals. The brain "sees" the image right side up.

SO... HOW DO WE SEE THEN?

In the retina are specialised receptor nerve cells, called rods and cones, which contain light-sensitive chemicals. The nerve cells get their names because of their shapes. The rods are about 1/400 of an inch (0.06 millimeters) long and about 1/100 of an inch (0.25 millimeters) thick.

The cones are shorter and thicker. There are about 120 million rod cells in each eye. They can work in dim light and are used for seeing black and white. The cone cells number about 7 million in each eye and function in full light. They provide colour vision. The cones contain a pigment known as visual purple or rhodopsin, which, it is believed, is broken down and bleached by light. This breaking down process sets off an electrical charge, which transmits the light in the form of nervous impulses to the brain by way of the optic nerve. These impulses are interpreted by the visual cortex to give us the sensation of sight. Colour blindness is due to defects in the cone cells.

Different cones are sensitive to different colours, so that a colour-blind person may be able to perceive some colours but not others. Colour blindness is inherited and rarely occurs in women.

Proper nutrition is important to preserve good eyesight. The rod and cone cells use a form of vitamin A to help convert light into nerve signals. The vitamin combines with proteins to make a light-sensitive chemical in the rods and colour sensitive chemicals in the cones. People who are get too little vitamin A do not see well at night.

GLAUCOMA

Glaucoma is the name given to a group of eye conditions in which the optic nerve is damaged at the point where it leaves the eye. Most commonly it is a rise in the pressure within the eye – intra-ocular pressure – that causes damage to the ocular structure. Intra-ocular pressure is determined by the balance between the rate of production and the rate of drainage of the aqueous fluid. In some cases the eye pressure is within the normal limits, but damage occurs due to a weakness in the optic nerve. In most cases both factors are involved in varying degrees with characteristic defects in the patient's sight.

SIGNS & SYMPTOMS OF GLAUCOMA

Chronic glaucoma often produces no symptoms – the gradual loss of vision goes unnoticed until total blindness results in some cases. Acute glaucoma happens more rapidly and varies in severity of pain, from a dull ache to severe pains in and around the eyes. Headache and fogging of vision is common and nausea and vomiting can occur – with a general feeling of being unwell.

On observation the eye may be red and swollen; the pupil can be fixed, semi-dilated and even oval in shape. Photophobia is common and at an early stage the patient may complain of seeing haloes or rainbow rings around lights at night.

CONVENTIONAL TREATMENT FOR GLAUCOMA

There is no "cure" for glaucoma, but it can be controlled. Even when treatment is effective, people with glaucoma need to have their eyes checked regularly, and often need to continue treatment for the rest of their lives.

Treatment for glaucoma focuses on lowering intraocular pressure (IOP) to a level the ophthalmologist thinks is unlikely to cause further optic nerve damage. This level is sometimes known as the "target pressure."

TYPES OF MEDICATIONS

If you have open-angle glaucoma (the most common type) the usual medication is for lowering intraocular pressure (IOP).

Miotics increase the outflow of aqueous (liquid) from the eye. These include:

IsoptoCarpine

- Ocusert
- Pilocar
- Pilopine

Epinephrine compounds also increase the outflow of aqueous from the eye.

Beta-blockers can reduce the amount of aqueous produced in the eye. These include:

Betagan

- Betimol
- Betoptic
- Ocupress
- Optipranalol
- Timoptic

Oral medication can also help control IOP. The most common oral medications are carbonic anhydrase inhibitors, which work to slow production of aqueous fluid in the eye. These pills include Daranide, Diamox and Neptazane.

POSSIBLE SIDE EFFECTS

Any medication, including eye drops, may have side effects. Some people taking glaucoma medication may experience:

- Stinging or redness of eyes
- Blurred vision
- Headache
- Changes in pulse, heartbeat or breathing
- Changes in sexual desire
- Mood changes
- Tingling of fingers and toes

- Drowsiness
- Loss of appetite
- Change of iris colour (in people with light-coloured eyes taking prostaglandin analogs).

HOMŒOPATHIC TREATMENT

Homœopathic treatment for glaucoma is, of course, a possibility and the following table lists some useful remedies:

Remedy	Comments
Gelsemium	One of the principle remedies in glaucoma – may be used more than any other. Certainly this has proved most valuable clinically. Pupils dilated and insensible to light, sore, red and aching. Bruised feeling in the back of the orbits, with pain travelling towards the occiput.
Aconite	Acute remedy. Sensation of heat, bloodshot eye, pain, sensation as if the eye were pushed out. Eyes hot, dry, sensitive to air. Fever, restlessness, < night.
Bryonia	Useful in the early stages, eye feels pressed out, sharp shooting pains And, of course, eyes are sore to move. Halo around lights, swollen lids.
Belladonna	Good for severe pains of glaucoma with throbbing headache and flushed face. Hot, dry eyes, photosensitive. Dilated pupils, immovable with burning heat.
Phosphorus	Eyeballs feel large and stiff; sensation as if something were pulled tightly over the eyes. Green and/or red haloes around lights. Loss of sight, darting pains.
Osmium	Sudden sharp pains; rainbow haloes or green colours around lights. Dim sight and photophobia.
Prunus spin	Bursting sensation, severe crushing pains. Worse on the right side, < touch, < pressure.
Jaborandi	Pupils contracted – do not react to light. Staring eyes, smarting pain in eyes. Worse on the left side.

Other remedies to consider include *Apis*, *Spigelia*, *Rhus tox*, *Colocynthis*, *Asafoetida*, *Opium* and *Sulphur*.

THE EYE

BLEPHARITIS

Blepharitis is the most frequent eye diagnosis in general practice. Blepharitis, in simple terms, is an inflammation of the eyelids.

SIGNS AND SYMPTOMS

Gritty burning sensation in the eyes and eyelids.

- On awakening, lid margins are swollen, red, irregular, and crusted.
- Red eyes.
- Watering or dry eyes.
- Difficult to open the eyes in the morning due to agglutination.

ASSOCIATED FACTORS

Adults over 60.

- Medical history of seborrheic dematitis of the scalp and other body parts.
- Exposure to chemical or environmental irritants.
- Crowded or unsanitary living conditions.
- Poor nutrition.
- Immunosuppression due to illness or medication.
- Diabetes mellitus.
- Acne rosacea.

This disease most frequently exists in elderly patients and can co-exist with poor tear production. It may be undetected by conventional medicine, so we should look out for it in practice.

CONVENTIONAL TREATMENT

As this is seen as an 'infective disease' the majority of conventional treatment is aimed at cleaning the affected area. If the Blepharitis is infective and/or has caused conjunctivitis to occur, then antibiotic cream is used additionally. If there is a systemic underlying cause (ie. seborrhoeic eczema – eczema produced by excessive excretion of sebum), then this will be treated with steroid medication.

HOMŒOPATHIC TREATMENT

This table shows the main remedies, also consider *Sulphur, Psorinum* and *Natrum mur.*

Remedy	Comments
Graphites	For chronic and acute conditions. Can be used in potency or topically (mother tincture in Vaseline) Particularly useful if the patient has seborrhoeic eczema. Burning and dryness – pale lids.

Mercurius sol	Syphilitic patients; ulcerated, thick, swollen lid margins. Especially the upper lids. Aching of the eyes.
Hepar sulph	Chronic blepharitis with ulcers and swelling of lids. Thick honeycomb scabs. Throbbing stinging pains.
Pulsatilla	Acute and chronic – tendency to formation of styes or abscesses.
Calcarea carb	Loss of eyelashes, thick discharge. Sensation of sand in the eye.
Arsenicum alb	Thick, red, excoriating lids. Burning lacrimation. Useful in the early stages of ulceration.
Staphysagria	Hard nodules on the eyelids, destruction of hair follicles. Itching and smarting.
Borax	Crusty and sticky eyelids. Eyelashes turn inwards and the lids become inflamed and 'cut against the eyeball.' (Murphy)

CATARACTS

The word cataract is used to describe the natural lens that has turned cloudy. Cataracts are not a disease, but rather a condition affecting the eye. As the natural lens of the eye becomes cloudy, it does not allow light to pass through it as well as it did when it was transparent. Cataracts usually start as a slight cloudiness that progressively grows more opaque. They are usually white, but may take on colour such as yellow or brown.

As the cataract becomes more mature (increasingly opaque and dense), the retina receives less and less light. The light that does reach the retina becomes increasingly blurred and distorted. This causes gradual impairment of vision. If left untreated, cataracts can cause blindness.

The development of cataracts is a normal part of the aging process, but they can result for a number of other reasons. Cataracts due to aging are a result of natural changes in the lens that coincide with other changes in the body. Traumatic cataracts may result from an injury or blow to the eye. Other causes of cataracts include the use of certain drugs or medications, exposure to harmful chemicals or excessive sun light, and some diseases. Some infants are born with congenital cataracts. In some cases, cataracts may even develop during childhood.

SIGNS AND SYMPTOMS OF A CATARACT

When there is only a hint of cloudiness to the lens, the cataract is classified as "trace." As the cloudiness progresses, the cataract may be classified as "mild" to "moderate." Once the cloudiness becomes very pronounced, the cataract is classified as "mature."

Vision with a cataract is similar to peering through a dirty or frost covered window. As the dirt or frost on the window increases, it becomes more difficult to see a clear image. As the cataract grows more opaque, images become less recognizable. Ultimately, the cataract may become so dense that it blocks light from entering the eye, resulting in needless blindness.

COMMON SYMPTOMS

- A gradual deterioration in vision over time.
- Objects may appear yellow, hazy, blurred or distorted.
- Vision at night or in low light conditions may be dramatically reduced.
- Vision in bright light or in the sunshine may be difficult due to glare.
- Halos may appear around bright lights at night.

CONVENTIONAL TREATMENT

Of all the fields of medicine, cataract surgery has been one of the greatest beneficiaries from advances in techniques and technology. Not so long ago, cataract surgery involved lengthy delays marked by deteriorating vision while the cataract "ripened," an extended and confining recovery period, plus the need for unsightly "cataract" glasses or contact lenses to achieve functional vision after surgery. Now, the surgery is a simple, outpatient procedure.

Modern advances in microsurgical techniques permit cataracts to be removed safely. An artificial lens can be implanted at the same time as the cataract is removed to provide a convenient means of restoring, and even enhancing, vision.

HOMŒOPATHIC TREATMENT

Treatment of cataract is usually a slow process. Burnett says that he expects to be successful, but that it may take many months or even years. Remedies to consider would include some of the 'Calcarea's' – *Calc carb, Calc fluor, Calc phos* and *Calc sulph* as well as *Magnesium carb, Phosphorus, Silica* and *Sulphur*. To differentiate (rather crudely) between the Calcarea's see the table below:

Remedy	Features
Calc carb	Sensation of cold in the eyes. Pain < reading or candle light. Tearful in the open air. Quivering eyelids. Pupils dilated.
Calc fluor	Sparks in front of the eyes. Flickering of vision. Ache in the eyeballs > pressing them tightly.
Calc phos	A feeling as if something was in the eye. Light hurts. Tearful when yawning.
Calc sulph	They can see only half an object. Protrusion of eyes. Purulent discharge.

CONJUNCTIVITIS

The conjunctiva is a thin, transparent mucus membrane covering the sclera or white of the eye and lining the upper and lower lids. It provides a protective covering to the eyeball and has a very rich blood supply. Conjunctivitis is the name given when this layer becomes inflamed. Due to its rich blood supply this layer on the white of the eye appears red or pinkish in colour, hence 'pink eye' being the common term. Conjunctivitis is a common eye condition and is usually self-limiting. It is caused by many different organisms, which bring about slightly different symptoms:

SIGNS AND SYMPTOMS

- Red eyes, often bilateral, but with one eye being more affected than the other one.
- Grittiness, as if something is in the eye.
- Watering with a discharge, varying from clear and watery, to profuse and thick, which can be green/yellow in colour.
- Itching and burning.
- Photophobia can be present. (Note – photophobia combined with visual loss may indicate iritis – refer if suspected.)
- Typically there is conjunctival infection, particularly where the conjunctiva folds over itself in the lower and upper lids.
- Discharge is variable but typically is present in the mornings, and on waking the eye is difficult to open as the eyelids are stuck together.
- The eyelids can look red and inflamed.
- Swelling may be present caused by damaged vessels leaking plasma into the tissue causing oedema, when this happens it is called chemosis.

CHRONIC VERNAL CONJUNCTIVITIS

This is less common than the hay fever type and is mainly seen in the spring or early summer, though some patients will present symptoms all year round in its chronic form. It usually affects the 10-14 year age group, boys more than girls, especially with a history of eczema, asthma and hay fever. The eyes feel gritty, water a lot, and produce a ropy discharge. The characteristic feature here is seen under the eyelid, with a distinctive 'cobblestone' appearance due to swelling of the *papillae* in the conjunctiva lining the upper lid.

SUBCONJUNCTIVAL HAEMORRHAGE

This follows a rupture of one of the capillaries and spreads a layer of blood across the sclera. This usually disappears after a week or so and is not important pathologically.

TRACHOMA

This is a chlamydial conjunctivitis that is rare in the UK, but is the most common cause of blindness worldwide.

ALLERGIC CONJUNCTIVITIS

Usually hay fever; with characteristic watery discharge, itching, sneezing, and catarrh – we'll have to treat this as part of a syndrome, but it may be, for some patients, the most important component.

PTERYGIUM

This is an opaque triangular encroachment seen on the nasal side of the eyeball crossing the conjunctiva. It is a degenerative change in the conjunctiva and is usually seen in dry, sunny countries and therefore possibly due to UV light. As long as it doesn't cross the cornea the only significance is cosmetic.

CONVENTIONAL TREATMENT

This is aimed at the type of causative factor involved. For bacterial conjunctivitis antibiotics are used, either as eye drops, cream, or systemically in tablet form. Both methods can be used together depending on the severity.

If the cause is due to Chlamydia then any sexual partners will need to be treated with oral antibiotics as well. When it is caused by a virus the use of topical steroids is employed in severe inflammation, but only if herpes simplex is excluded. Unfortunately it is common to have rebound inflammation once the steroid eye drops have been stopped. Antibiotic cover is sometimes given to control any secondary infection.

For allergic responses antihistamine tablets are given with mast cell stabilising eye drops. Topical steroids are required in severe cases but long-term use is avoided if possible because of the possibility of steroid-induced glaucoma or cataract.

In sudden onset allergies, found commonly in children who have been playing in fields of long grass or hay in the summer, the swelling is generally a lot better by the time they have reached the GP or hospital. The patient is not treated medically, but advised to lie down with eyes closed and apply a cold compress, and to avoid the causative factor if known.

HOMŒOPATHIC TREATMENT

Conjunctivitis, though not a sight-threatening disease, can cause a great deal of misery and suffering to the patient, especially when it lasts throughout the summer, as in the allergic hay fever type conjunctivitis. In these allergic type cases the constitutional picture may be obscured due to the predominant symptoms present and, as with any complaint, it is useful to see which are the most important symptoms at that time needing treatment. For example: a distraught mother phones you about her son who, after playing in a field, has suddenly developed a swollen red eye which appears to look like a large water blister on the inside of his eyelid, with the only modalities being, better for cold application and worse for touch. The swelling is the main symptom and combined with the two modalities given, *Apis* is the remedy indicated. Then once the presenting complaint has subsided, the patient's constitutional level can be addressed.

HOMŒOPATHIC REMEDY DIFFERENTIATION (CONJUNCTIVITIS)

Useful places to look if in doubt include: Dr. A Norton's Book, "Ophthalmic Diseases and Therapeutics" and "The Best of Burnett".

EUPHRASIA

Euphrasia is especially indicated in the first acute stages, and is caused by exposure to cold. The discharge is profuse, thick and yellow, making the lids sore and excoriated. Intolerance to light is usually present with the conjunctiva looking red and Chemosis may even be present (Chemosis is an oedematous swelling of the conjunctiva). Concomitant symptoms are great irritability with a watery nasal discharge and sneezing.

Whether the condition is caused by an infection, allergy or contact lens cleaner, 10 drops of *Euphrasia* mother tincture to 0.25 litre of warm water, every 4 hours, is very soothing.

PULSATILLA

This is one of our most important remedies in catarrhal and purulent conjunctivitis. The discharges are thick, bland, yellow and profuse, with the conjunctiva becoming irritated and the lids itch and burn, compelling the patient to rub. All of these symptoms are ameliorated in fresh air and aggravated in a warm room. *Sulphur* has similar itching and burning, but the itching starts in the morning and continues all day, while *Pulsatilla* is worse in the evening and ameliorated by bathing (*Sulphur* is aggravated by bathing).

Both Norton and Murphy mention its use in treating Ophthalmia neonatorum (a form of conjunctivitis which affects newborn infants), with Norton using it as an inter-current remedy during treatment with *Arg nit*. Both *Pulsatilla* and *Arg nit* are important anti-sycotic remedies.

ARGENTUM NITRICUM

Norton describes this as one of his most serviceable remedies in the whole Materia Medica for any form of purulent inflammation of the conjunctiva. Murphy writes: "violent painful purulent Ophthalmia, with great swelling of the conjunctiva (Chemosis) and indicated in Ophthalmia neonatorum".

The absence of subjective symptoms, with the profuse purulent discharge, and the swollen lids or conjunctiva, indicates this remedy alone. The inflammatory symptoms usually subside in the open air and are aggravated in a warm room, with eye symptoms being worse when abdominal symptoms are present.

APIS

Apis is indicated in any form of conjunctivitis where there are swollen, red, oedematous eyelids or conjunctiva (Chemosis). The character of the pains, which are stinging and shooting, is an important indication, and serve to distinguish between this remedy and *Rhus tox*, as both are very similar, but *Rhus tox* has the opposite modalities to *Apis*. All of the symptoms are worse for heat and evening time and better for cold application. Often concomitant symptoms such as drowsiness and absence of thirst are present.

NUX VOMICA

This remedy has been proven of special value in Vernal conjunctivitis (Spring catarrh) where there is excessive photophobia, lacrymation and morning aggravation of all symptoms. The pains are characteristically sharp and darting or burning in and around the eyes, and are sometimes relieved by bathing the eyes in cold water. The gastric symptoms of *Nux vom* are often present.

KALI BICHROMICUM

This is also indicated in Vernal conjunctivitis (Spring catarrh) especially when there are characteristic symptoms of ropy discharge and when the lids are granular in appearance. There is only moderate irritation of the eye, and little or no photophobia or redness present. The eye is sensitive to touch but not painful otherwise. Useful in chronic cases.

ARSENICUM

Arsenicum is used where there is profuse, watery, burning discharge, as in a cold, influenza and similar cases. There is intense photophobia and swelling of the conjunctiva and area around the eye. Also a sensation of sand in the eyes and it is said that the conjunctiva can look like 'raw beef'. The eyelids can also feel dry and as if they are rubbing against the eyeballs. Concomitant symptoms generally are restlessness and thirst for small quantities of water.

BELLADONNA

Belladonna is for the early stages of conjunctivitis where there is swelling and the eye looks red, puffy and shiny. There is usually a great sense of dryness with smarting and burning pains in the eye. Photophobia is marked and concomitant symptoms are headaches with a red face and a dry fever.

MERCURIUS

This is one of the best remedies in gonorrhoeal or purulent conjunctivitis, in either acquired or hereditary syphilitic subjects. The discharge can be profuse or scanty, both burning and excoriating with marked photophobia, which is worse for heat and glare of the fire.

It is indicated in chronic conjunctivitis from taking cold and where the lids are stuck together in the morning on waking. Concomitant symptoms of snuffles, bone pain, restlessness and all symptoms being worse at night are important when selecting this remedy.

AMBROSIA

Ambrosia is well indicated in the allergic hay fever conjunctivitis with lacrymation and intolerable itching of the eyelids, which burn and smart. Concomitant symptoms are sneezing with watery coryza that can feel cold.

Other remedies of note are:

Sulphur, Aconite, Rhus tox, Sepia, Arnica, Calendula, Kali iod, Calc carb, Calc sulph, Alumina, Chamomilla, Ipecacuanha, Allium cepa, Borax and *Hydrophyllum.*

UVEITIS

Crudely put, the eye is shaped much like a tennis ball, hollow inside with three different layers of tissue surrounding a central cavity. The outermost is the sclera (white coat of the eye) and the innermost is the retina, image-gathering tissue in the back of the eye. The middle layer between the sclera and retina is called the uvea, from the Greek word "uva" meaning grape. In the laboratory, it looks much like a "peeled grape." When the uvea becomes inflamed, the condition is called Uveitis.

The uvea contains many of the blood vessels that nourish the eye. Inflammation of the uvea can affect the cornea, the retina, the sclera, and other vital parts of the eye. Since the uvea borders many important parts of the eye, inflammation of this layer may be sight-threatening and more serious than the more common inflammations of the outside layers of the eye.

SIGNS AND SYMPTOMS

Uveitis may come on suddenly with redness and pain, or it may be slow in onset with little pain or redness, but gradual blurring of vision. When the uvea is inflamed near the front of the eye in the iris, it is described as iritis. If the uvea is inflamed in the middle of the eye involving the ciliary body, it is called cyclitis. If the inflammation is in the back of the eye affecting the choroid, it is called choroiditis. Uveitis has many different causes. It may result from a virus (such as shingles, mumps, or herpes), a fungus (such as histoplasmosis), or a parasite (such as toxoplasmosis). In most cases, the cause remains unknown.

Uveitis can also be related to disease in other parts of the body (such as arthritis) or come as a consequence of injury to the eye. Inflammation in one eye can result from a severe injury to the opposite eye (sympathetic Uveitis). A careful eye examination by an ophthalmologist is extremely important when symptoms occur. Inflammations inside the eye can permanently affect sight, and at times, lead to blindness.

CONVENTIONAL TREATMENT

Prompt treatment is necessary to minimise any loss of vision. Eye drops, especially steroids and pupil dilators, are medications used to reduce inflammation and pain. For deeper inflammation, oral medication or injections may be necessary. Complications such as glaucoma (high pressure in the eye), cataracts (clouding of the lens of the eye), or new blood vessel formation (neovascularization), also may need treatment in the course of the disease. If complications are advanced, conventional surgery or laser surgery may be necessary. Uveitis arising in the front or middle part of the eye (iritis or cyclitis) is commonly more sudden in onset, generally lasting six to eight weeks, and in the early stages can usually be controlled by the frequent use of drops. Often, this type of Uveitis cannot be given a specific cause. Uveitis in the back part of the eye (choroiditis) is commonly slower in onset and may last longer, and is often more difficult to treat.

HOMŒOPATHIC TREATMENT

You won't find Uveitis in Murphy's Repertory, so you have to do some detective work. Essentially, if you go for 'inflammation' (p. 544) and move on from there, you won't go far wrong. You can expect the usual suspects to be helpful; *Apis, Arsenicum, Belladonna, Rhus tox, Mercury*, and so forth. Topical treatments as ever may help – with *Euphrasia* being the number one topical (and/or potentised) remedy.

SQUINT

Under normal circumstances the newborn baby learns to focus his/her eyes on an object within a few weeks. During the learning process the eyes wander independently – eventually learning to operate together to attain binocular vision. However, if one of the eyes is not functioning properly for any reason, there may be two separate points of focus, causing double vision. The confusion this causes is rectified by the brain suppressing the information from one (the weaker) of the eyes. That eye then becomes 'lazy' or amblyopic (dim) and gradually ceases to function at all. The suppression continues over the next few years and by age five the child is left with monocular vision. The major consequence of this is usually cosmetic in that the lazy eye will not always follow the direction of gaze.

CONVENTIONAL TREATMENT

The usual treatment is to cover the good eye with a patch to encourage macular vision in the weak eye, and if necessary to operate on the muscles of the lazy eye to bring it in line with the other.

Sudden squints which happen in adults are likely to be due to damage to one to the nerves which supply the extrinsic muscles of the eye – possible causes include: diabetes, MS, tumour, or aneurysm compressing the nerve.

HOMŒOPATHIC TREATMENT

This is not an easy condition to treat. It is often of very long standing and may even have been adapted to. Remedies to consider would certainly include *Belladonna, Cicuta virosa, Cyclamen,* and *Natrum mur*. Given that this may be a problem that dates from very early age, I would also consider a miasmatic remedy, possibly *Syphilinum*.

LACRIMAL PATHOLOGY

STICKY EYE

This can be seen shortly after birth and is caused by a narrowing of the tear ducts, which may not fully develop for three or four months at which point the problem will spontaneously remit. While the problem is present, the tears will flow down the cheeks, but at night they can form a stagnant pool that evaporates and then thickens. This causes the eyelids to stick and/or infect. Treatment consists of cleaning and massage of the lacrimal duct.

EPIPHORA

This is a similar condition that occurs in adults, which can be caused by failure of the lacrimal ducts to approximate to the eyeball. This can be caused by atrophy of the tissues or by a cyst.

SJORGEN'S SYNDROME

This is atrophy of the lacrimal glands leading to loss of secretions and consequent grittiness, itching, and recurrent inflammation of the conjunctiva. It is associated with rheumatoid arthritis and there can be accompanying dryness of the salivary glands.

HOMŒOPATHIC TREATMENT

Treatment of any lacrimal problem can always start with the topical, and no remedy is finer than *Euphrasia*. Applied directly to the eye as diluted tincture this is a fabulous remedy, nearly always being at least palliative. For addressing the underlying pathology in Sticky eye and Epiphora I would choose from *Natrum mur*, *Petroleum*, *Fluoric acid*, and *Silica*. The latter often being the first choice remedy. For Sjorgen's syndrome the pathology may be both deep and systemic and some of the remedies covered as helpful for rheumatism in the musculoskeletal chapter would be highly appropriate.

EYELID PATHOLOGY

MEIBOMIAN/TARSAL CYSTS

The centre of the eyelids are strengthened by a plate of connective tissue, the Tarsus. Within the Tarsus are small glands whose function is to secrete sebaceous fluid that lubricates the lids. If these glands get infected they tend to enlarge and form what are known as Meibomian cysts (which aren't actually cysts – ie. blocked ducts – but just these swellings). The swollen reddened glands are known as Chalazion ('collection of rubble') and cause watering and irritation. They can be easily differentiated from styes by their position – halfway up the lid. *Hepar sulph* and *Silica* are both good 'first-choice' remedies.

STYE

The stye or hordeolum (hordeum = barley) is an infection of the root of an eyelash. This produces an inflamed swelling with a yellow head frequently containing staphylococci. The classic number one choice of remedy is *Staphysagria*, and I've found it to be fabulously effective.

PTOSIS

This is a falling of the lids, due to paralysis of the muscles. It is frequently a congenital disease (present since birth) although it can occur in old age…being senile ptosis; and is then due to atrophy of the tissues. *Gelsemium, Alumina* and *Sepia* are frequently effective, indicated remedies.

CORNEAL PATHOLOGY

ARCUS SENILIS

This is a lesion of the outer edge of the cornea (thicker at the top or bottom) which indicates an abnormally high amount of lipid in the blood (lipid is a fat-like substance – like cholesterol) – therefore this is indicative of vascular pathology. It never extends far enough into the cornea to affect sight.

KERATITIS

This is the name given to an infection of the cornea. The cornea is not the usual target for bacterial invasion (with the exception of gonococcus) therefore most infections are viral. Bacteria can easily invade the cornea when there is already some damage. It is for this reason that any corneal abrasions must be observed very closely to make sure that the little blighters don't invade resulting in a corneal ulcer. The cornea can also be damaged by drying – possibly as a feature of Sjorgen's Syndrome, by Trachoma (severe and prolonged inflammation of the membrane lining the eyelids), or by the failure of the lids to meet in thyrotoxicosis. Acne rosacea can cause keratitis in some people, but the problem should resolve as the skin condition improves.

HERPES SIMPLEX KERATITIS

This is a cold sore that occurs on the cornea. This will take the form of either tiny pinhead dots or of a ragged branching ulcer; the latter is known as a dendtritic ulcer. It will be very painful with photophobia and reddening of the sclera.

HERPES ZOSTER – SHINGLES

Shingles may also affect the cornea if it is occurring on the ophthalmic nerve. A blistering rash will be seen on the forehead and down the side of the nose. This is most likely to affect elderly patients causing pain along the site of the nerve and it can be very persistent.

HOMŒOPATHIC TREATMENT

For both of the herpetic conditions I would recommend *Rhus tox* as the top remedy. For corneal problems in general there often seems to be a need for *Calcarea carb*, if that doesn't seem to fit the case sufficiently well, other remedies to include *Cannabis indica*, and *Pulsatilla*. As for many eye conditions, liberal doses of *Euphrasia* tincture can really help with any immediate symptoms as well as aiding the work of deeper remedies.

FURTHER READING

R L Gregory **Eye and Brain – The Psychology of Seeing**
BAS Printers Ltd. *ISBN 297-77303-8*

Ian Watson **The Tao of Homeopathy**
Cutting Edge Publications, *ISBN 0-9517657-2-8*

Dr Douglas Gibson **Studies of Homœopathic Remedies**
Beaconsfield, *ISBN 0-906584-17-5*

Nancy Herrick **Animal Mind, Human Voices**
Hahnemann Clinic Publishing, *ISBN 0-9635368-1-8*

J Ellis Barker **The Story Of My Eyes**
B Jain Publishers, *ISBN 81-8056-502-5*

NOTES

CONTENTS

THE AUDITORY SYSTEM

THE STRUCTURE OF THE EAR

Like the ears of other mammals, the human ear consists of three sections: the outer, middle, and inner ear. The outer and middle ears function only for hearing, while the inner ear also serves the functions of balance and orientation.

The outer ear is made up of the auricle, or pinna, and the outer auditory canal. The auricle is the curved part of the ear attached to the side of the head by small ligaments and muscles. It consists largely of elastic cartilage, and its shape helps collect sound waves from the air. The earlobe, or lobule, which hangs from the lower part of the auricle, contains mostly fatty tissue.

The outer auditory canal, which measures about 3 cm (about 1.25 in) in length, is a tubular passageway lined with delicate hairs and small glands that produce a wax-like secretion called cerumen. The canal leads from the auricle to a thin taut membrane – the eardrum or tympanic membrane, which is nearly round in shape and about 10 mm wide.

The cerumen in the outer auditory canal traps and retains dust and dirt that might otherwise end up on the eardrum, impairing its ability to vibrate.

The inner two-thirds of the outer auditory canal is housed by the temporal bone, which also surrounds the middle and inner ear. The temporal bone protects these fragile areas of the ear.

The eardrum separates the outer ear from the middle ear. A narrow passageway called the eustachian tube connects the middle ear to the throat and the back of the nose. The eustachian tube helps keep the eardrum intact by equalizing the pressure between the middle and outer ear. When we yawn or swallow, the eustachian tube opens, and some of the air in the middle ear passes into the throat, adjusting the pressure in the middle ear to match the pressure in the outer ear… well, in theory at least. This equalizing of pressure on both sides of the eardrum prevents it from rupturing.

The middle ear is a narrow, air-filled chamber that extends vertically for about 15 mm and for nearly the same distance horizontally. Inside this chamber is a linked chain of three ossicles, or very small bones. Both the Latin and common names of these bones are derived from their shapes. They are called the malleus, or hammer; the incus, or anvil; and the stapes, or stirrup, which is the tiniest bone in the body, being smaller than a grain of rice.

THE INNER EAR

The chain of bones in the middle ear leads into the convoluted structures of the inner ear, or labyrinth, which contains organs of both hearing and balance. The three main structures of the inner ear are the cochlea, the vestibule, and the three semicircular canals. The vestibule helps the body maintain balance and orientation by monitoring the sensations of movement and position.

Most of the pathology of the external auditory canal is that of the skin which lines it. It is so warm and moist that some patients are prone to chronic eczema, with itchy discharge and often with small blisters.

Cleaning the ear with small instruments can abrade the area and lead to periodic infections – these can be painful.

OTITIS EXTERNA (OUTER EAR)

This can occur after swimming in dirty water, and consists of a fungus that produces a cheesy discharge. Placing small objects in the ear – not a course of action that I recommend – can also cause it.

OTITIS MEDIA (MIDDLE EAR)

This is one of the commonest childhood complaints and is due to a blockage of the Eustachian Tube at the lower end, probably on account of enlarged adenoids or catarrh. If a cold or other respiratory tract infection occurs this may 'back up' into the middle ear and cause pain – of a throbbing or stabbing nature. The secretions can easily become infected with streptococci or staphylococci and the drum can burst with all the pressure, and with all the pressure pushing it outward, the drum can eventually burst (and fortunately then relieve the pain). Even when the drum doesn't burst there can still be some trauma – causing it to look like crazy paving – but this should heal easily.

CONVENTIONAL TREATMENT

The conventional approach to treating otitis media is based on the use of antibiotics, although increasingly there are concerns that these are becoming ineffective in children (and adults). Consequently the emphasis is starting to shift to preventative treatments – various factors seem to predispose a child to otitis media and the following are generally acknowledged as catalysts worth avoiding if possible:

- Contact with large numbers of children
- Use of formula milk
- Use of a dummy
- Passive smoking

For some suitable remedies take a look at the following table. These remedies can be helpful in otitis media, and may be of use in other pathologies of the ear.

Remedy	Comments
Belladonna	Tearing pain in the middle or outer ear. Heat. Parotid glands swollen, very sensitive to loud tones – hearing VERY acute. Child cries out in sleep.
Calcarea carbonica	Throbbing, cracking in the ears, pulsating pain as if something would press out. Deafness from working in water. Enlargement of glands. Sensitive to cold around the ears and neck.
Calcarea sulphurica	Deafness with discharge of matter from the middle ear - sometimes mixed with blood. Pimples around the ear.
Chamomilla	Ringing in the ears. Earache with soreness and irritation. Swelling and heat drives the patient frantic. Stitching pain. Ears feel stopped up.
Hepar sulphuris	Discharge of fetid pus from the ears. Whizzing and throbbing in the ears. Useful for deafness following scarlet fever.
Kali bichromicum	Ears swollen with tearing pains. Thick yellow, fetid, sticky discharge. Sharp stitches in the left ear.
Lycopodium	Thick, yellow, offensive discharge. Eczema behind the ears. Humming and roaring with hardness of hearing. Every noise causes a peculiar echo in the ear.
Mercury	Fetid bloody discharge. Boils in the external canal.
Mercurius dulcis	This remedy has a marked effect on inflammation of the ear. Useful for eustachian catarrh and deafness. Closure of the eustachian canal.
Pulsatilla	Senasation as if something were being forced outwards, ears feel stuffed making hearing difficult. Thick bland discharge with offensive odour.
Silica	Roaring in the ears. Fetid discharge. Sensitive to noise.
Sulphur	Whizzing in the ears. Deafness preceded by extremely sensitive hearing. Catarrhal deafness.

GLUE EAR

The Eustachian Tube is normally full of air (as it is opened every time we swallow), thus enabling us to hear properly. If it gets full of fluid, however, speech and hearing can be impaired at a critical age. One in two hundred children will suffer from Glue Ear.

The mucus membrane of the middle ear normally secretes a small amount of mucus, but if the bottom end of the Eustachian Tube is plugged up (adenoids too big?) then the fluid builds up and stops proper hearing. Treatment is normally by inserting grommets in the drum – these allow the air to enter and the ossicles (ear bones) to vibrate freely.

OTOSCLEROSIS

This is a genetic disorder wherein the bones of the ear, especially the stapes (the 'last in the chain') get spongy and then harden. This impedes all vibration especially the higher tones and stops the dampening effect of the stapes – causing an odd effect whereby speech is better heard against a background of noise. The hearing loss is usually bilateral and treatment is by surgery, although small doses of *Calc fluor* may halt the degeneration.

MENIERE'S DISEASE (INNER EAR)

This is a combination of symptoms that can be particularly distressing. Patients suffer auditory symptoms of deafness, tinnitus and/or physical symptoms of vertigo and nausea.

Because the labyrinth (which controls balance) and the cochlea are so close together, they share the vestibulochlear nerve and that is probably why this particular set of symptoms are shared in Meniere's disease.

The disease is thought to be caused by a sudden increase in pressure in the labyrinth (for unknown reasons); the symptoms in full are:

- Sudden fluctuating loss of hearing and/or tinnitus
- Vertigo
- Nausea
- Sense of pressure in the ear

These symptoms occur periodically at frequencies from weekly to every few months. There is a tendency for symptoms to increase in frequency, intensity and duration over a period of years. This means that the patient can still be symptom-free for periods of time, however it has been noted that there is a general increase in the level of deafness/tinnitus, which is maintained between attacks.

Each attack can last for hours or days and will usually confine the patient to bed (mostly from the vertigo). For some odd reason there is a 'constitutional' type of person who is more prone to Meniere's – fair-haired, blue eyed, and between 30 and 60 years.

CONVENTIONAL TREATMENT

Medication is used to control the frequency of attacks or to reduce the feelings of nausea. There are also a range of exercises that can help with the vertigo – these are usually planned and explained by a physiotherapist or a hearing therapist. There is also evidence that a low salt diet can reduce both frequency and severity of the attacks of vertigo.

HOMŒOPATHIC TREATMENT

This is another one of those diseases that turn up in homœopathic clinics. Conventional medicine doesn't always offer sufferers all that they want, and so many try the 'complementary route' to alleviate their symptoms. Experience has shown homœopathy to be of great help to some patients. Here's a small selection of remedies that may be useful:

China sulph

Violent ringing, buzzing, and roaring in the ears with deafness

PHOSPHORUS

Difficulty in hearing – especially the human voice. Re-echoing of sounds. Dullness of hearing after typhoid.

NATRUM SALICYLICUM

Tinnitus of a low tone. Deafness, and auditory vertigo – I don't know that this could be used to 'conventionally' describe this condition (it's a phrase we find in some of our older Materia Medicas) but it perfectly describes Meniere's disease.

SANGUINARIA

Earache with accompanying headache. Burning in the ears. Humming and roaring. Polyps in the ear.

GLONOINE

Throbbing in the ears – each beat of the heart is heard in the ears, full sensation in the ears.

FURTHER READING

Dr. Noel Pratt **Homœopathic Prescribing**
Beaconsfield
ISBN 0-906584-03-:5

Madeleine Harland and Glen Finn **The Barefoot Homœopath**
Hyden House
ISBN 1-85623-001-5

John H Clarke **The Presciber**
Pitman Press
ISBN 0-85032-088-7

S P Koppikar **Clinical Experiences of 70 Years in Homœopathy**
B Jain Publishers
ISBN 81-8056-029-5

NOTES

NOTES